54027000348712

AF598640

PHARMACOLOGY OF ANXIOLYTIC DRUGS

WHO Expert Series on Neuroscience

WHO's Mental Health Programme has three major objectives which it hopes to achieve in cooperation with its Member States. These are, first, to prevent or control mental and neurological disorders and psychosocial problems; second, to ensure a broad utilization of mental health knowledge in general health care; and third, to help countries in dealing with psychosocial aspects of overall development.

The WHO Expert Series on Neuroscience, previous to 1995 called the WHO Expert Series on Biological Psychiatry, is intended to help mainly in the achievement of the first two of these objectives. It is one of the many efforts the Organization has undertaken to promote the exchange of information and collaborative research on mental and neurological disorders.

The themes for inclusion in the Series are selected by the Heads of the WHO Collaborating Centres for Research and Training in Mental Health and Neuroscience located in 34 countries, and the texts are produced by experts participating in the WHO programme.

Series Editors: J. Costa e Silva
L. L. Prilipko

Current Volumes

Vol. 1	Haag, H., Rüther, E., Hippius, H. *Tardive Dyskinesia*
Vol. 2	Grof, P., Akther, M.I., Campbell, M., Gottfries, C.G., Khan, I. Lampierre, Y., Lemberger, L., Müller-Örlinghausen, B., and Woggon, B. *Clinical Evaluation of Psychotropic Drugs for Psychiatric Disorders*
Vol. 3	Racagni, G., Masotto, C., Steardo, L. *Pharmacology of Anxiolytic Drugs*
Vol. 4	Tabakoff, B., Hoffman, P. (Eds) *Biological Aspects of Alcoholism*
Vol. 5	Maj, M., Starace, F., Sartorius, N. *Mental Disorders in HIV-1 Infection and AIDS*

Pharmacology of Anxiolytic Drugs

Giorgio Racagni, Claudio Masotto
and Luca Steardo

WHO Expert Series on Neuroscience
Volume 3

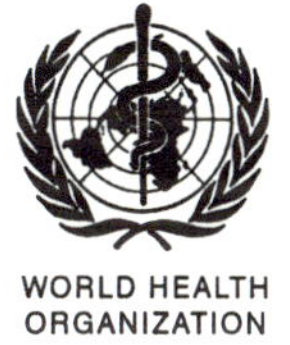

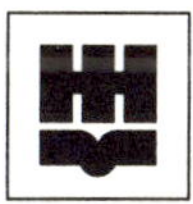

Hogrefe & Huber Publishers
Seattle • Toronto • Göttingen • Bern

Library of Congress Cataloging-in-Publication Data

Racagni, Giorgio

Pharmacology of anxiolytic drugs / Giorgio Racagni, Claudio Masotto, and Luca Steardo.

p. cm. — (WHO expert series on neuroscience: vol. 3)

Includes bibliographical references and index.

ISBN 0-88937-088-5

1. Tranquilizing drugs. I. Masotto, Claudio, 1956- . II. Steardo, Luca, 1947- . III. Title. IV. Series.

[DNLM: 1. Anti-Anxiety Agents — pharmacology. 2. Anxiety Disorders — drug therapy. W1 WH48 v.3 / QV 77.9 R118p 1997]

RM333.R33 1997

615'.7882 — dc20

DNLM/DLC

For Library of Congress 96-32870

Canadian Cataloguing in Publication Data

Racagni, Giorgio

Pharmacology of anxiolytic drugs

(WHO expert series on neuroscience: v. 3)

Includes bibliographical references and index.

ISBN 0-88937-088-5

1.Tranquilizing drugs. I. Masotto, Claudio, 1956- II. Steardo, Luca, 1947- III. World Health Organization. IV. Title. V. Series.

RM333.R.33 1997 615/.7882 C96-990002-3

USA: P.O. Box 2487, Kirkland, WA 98083-2487
Phone (206) 820-1500, Fax (206) 823-8324
CANADA: 12 Bruce Park Avenue, Toronto, Ontario M4P 2S3
Phone (416) 482-6339
GERMANY: Rohnsweg 25, D-37085 Göttingen
Phone +49 551 496090, Fax +49 551 4960988
SWITZERLAND: Länggass-Strasse 76, CH-3000 Bern 9
Phone +41 31 300-4500, Fax +41 31 300 4590

Printed in the United States of America

ISBN 0-88937-088-5

Hogrefe & Huber Publishers

Seattle • Toronto • Göttingen • Bern

CONTENTS

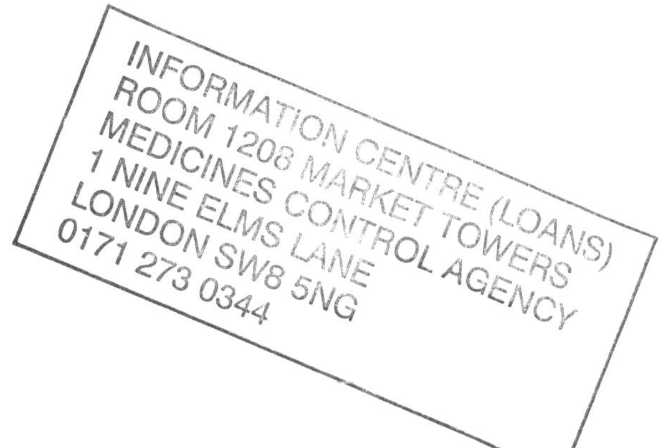

Group II — Compounds with Benzodiazepine-like Activity

Group III — Compounds Acting on Non-Benzodiazepine Receptors

Group IV — Other Compounds

INTRODUCTION

Since ancient times man has searched for the means to allay his everyday worries, relieve feelings of inner anxiety and facilitate a restful sleep.

Ethanol was the first agent used to ease tension, and today it is still widely prescribed for the relief of anxiety — but inappropriately so, since its therapeutic value is limited and its chronic ingestion is associated with deleterious effects.

In the second part of the last century, bromide salts and compounds similar in their effects to ethanol, such as paraldehyde and chloral hydrate, were introduced into medical practice as a sedative for the treatment of anxiety and related disorders. They were extensively prescribed, and became popular: and the fact that they were sold freely in many western countries promoted self medication and chronic ingestion. Unfortunately, it took over 50 years for the disadvantages of these drugs to become apparent. By the 1930s, it was well recognized that the bromides possess cumulative effects and provoke toxic delirium. Paraldehyde appeared to be prone to inducing psychotic states. These unwanted deleterious effects, together with their poor effectiveness, led to a decline in popularity and subsequent drastic decrease in their use.

Barbiturates replaced bromides and paraldehyde on clinicians' prescriptions, becoming the dominant antianxiety agents through the first half of this century. They had been introduced into human pharmacotherapy in the early 1900s. Long-acting barbiturates were extensively used despite their many side-effects, and only in the mid 1950s did considerable concern arise over their safety and efficacy as anxiolytics. It became evident that the anxiolytic effects of these agents were very non specific, occurring as part of generalized central nervous system (CNS) depression. Their clinical efficacy seemed questionable because most patients did not achieve relief of anxiety without coincident unwanted sedation, impairing intellectual and motor skills. As with previous sedatives, barbiturates offered considerable potential for abuse and addiction, as well as the hazards associated with overdosage, which occurred at doses not greatly exceeding the therapeutic range. This led to a growing dissatisfaction, which accelerated efforts to find safer and non sedating anxiolytic agents.

The first of the new drugs was meprobamate, a chemical variant of a weak and short-acting muscle relaxant, mephenesine. Early pharmacological reports stated that meprobamate was not sedative and emphasized that the drug had more specific antianxiety effects than barbiturates, because it might selectively affect brain systems modulating anxiety. However, further controlled studies failed to substantiate the initial claims and suggested that the differences between meprobamate and barbiturates were trivial, since meprobamate shared many of the unwanted properties of barbiturates, including excessive sedation, an impressive liability to induce physical dependence and occurrence of intoxication on overdosage.

The introduction, in the late 1950s, of benzodiazepines (BDZs) into medical practice produced a major impact on the pharmacological treatment of anxiety disorders. The BDZs rapidly became extremely popular with physicians and patients. Their success heralded the development of a whole range of other BDZs which is still being extended more than 30 years after the arrival of chlordiazepoxide. BDZs are currently the primary pharmacological agents used; and they do appear to be more effective, and certainly considerably safer than barbiturates or meprobamate. In fact, most patients experience satisfactory anxiolytic effects in doses that do not produce clinically important sedation or impairment of cognitive and motor functioning. Therefore, BDZs seemed to meet many of the requirements for an ideal antianxiety drug.

However, it is gradually becoming apparent that some patients develop a psychological and physical dependence. This has prompted efforts to develop new, effective anxiolytic agents lacking any propensity to induce dependence. Newer anxiolytic compounds have been developed recently which seem to have the anxiolytic properties of the BDZs, but fewer of the disadvantages. Some, such as cyclopyrrolones and imidazopyridines, which lack structural homology with the BDZ, act on or near to the BDZ receptors. Others are more innovative and do not affect the BDZ/gamma aminobutyric acid (GABA) receptor into the brain. In animal models, such agents appear inactive in terms of dependence, tolerance and abuse. Since they seem to possess similar efficacy to BDZ, with a pharmacological profile consistent with safety during long term use, these agents may constitute a significant alternative to previous pharmacotherapies for anxiety disorders.

Classification of Antianxiety Medications

Depending on their structural and functional features, antianxiety drugs may be divided into four groups:

- benzodiazepines
- compounds with benzodiazepine-like activity
- compounds acting on non benzodiazepine receptor sites
- other compounds.

The latter class of derivatives includes compounds with antianxiety properties, which however, are used mainly in different pathologies, for instance, tricyclic antidepressants and beta-blocking drugs.

Group I
Benzodiazepines

Benzodiazepine Structure

BDZs are so named because their core structure consists of a benzene ring fused to a 7-membered 1,4-diazepine ring.

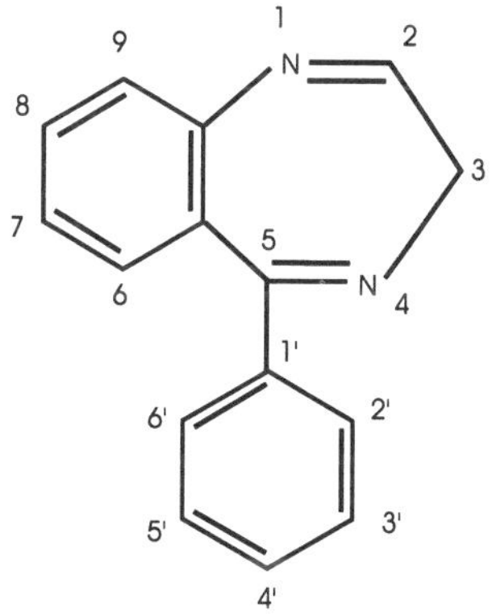

BDZ

Almost all BDZs also have a 5-aryl substituent ring. They differ in the chemical nature of the substituent groups at positions 1, 2, 3, 4, (of the diazepine ring), position 7 (of the benzene ring) and position 2' (of the 5-aryl substituent ring).

By manipulating the structure of the ring systems, medical chemists have produced a number of different compounds with a similar spectrum of pharmacologic activity including:

- 1,5-benzodiazepines
- 2,3-benzodiazepines
- thieno or pyrazolo diazepines in which the benzene ring is replaced with an heteroaromatic nucleus
- tiazolo and imidazolobenzodiazepines with tiazolo or imidazolo ring replaced at position 1 to 3
- 3-hydroxybenzodiazepines with the OH group located at position 3
- nitrobenzodiazepines with a NO_2 group at position 7
- cyclopropylbenzodiazepines with a ciclopropyl group linked to the nitrogen group at position 1.

Activity is increased by the substitution of electron withdrawing groups at position 7 and 2'; alkyl substituents larger than methyl at position 1 decreases activity. The replacement of the carbonyl function at position 2 with hydrogen, reduction of the N_4-C_5 double bond, or the introduction of halo-substituents at 3 or 4 position drastically reduce activity. The substitution of the aryl ring with a keto group at position 5 and the presence of a methyl group at 4 provide structural properties for the antagonism at BDZ modulatory site. Derivatives in a given subgroup are metabolized in the liver by a similar mechanism and therefore have half lives within the same broad ranges. However, even BDZs with very similar chemical structures can differ greatly in their potency, rate of adsorption and other important pharmacologic parameters.

Benzodiazepine Pharmacology

A careful evaluation of the pharmacologic properties of antianxiety agents is necessary for clinicians to address appropriate anxiolytic treatments. Several thousand "classic" BDZs have been synthesized, and more than 50 are at present available worldwide for medical use.

Although there are many similarities among the various BDZ compounds, there are also significant differences. It has been widely accepted that these agents are virtually identical pharma-codinamically, with pharmacokinetic factors accounting for the clinical important differences among them. Large quantitative variations in the intrinsic affinity for the receptor sites require appropriate adjustment of dosage in order to compare the clinical activity of various BDZs. After this adjustment, it is difficult to distinguish substantial qualitative differences in the character of their clinical action. Therefore, pharmacokinetic factors, particularly those that characterize onset and duration of action, are the main reasons why particular BDZ may be recommended for particular clinical applications.

However, the advent of the new drugs, both BDZs and non BDZs, which act as a partial agonist at BDZ receptors, seems to make it possible to separate — independently of pharmacokinetic differences — the anxiolytic, sedative, anticonvulsant effects. The correct use of BDZ anxiolytics therefore needs a knowledge of pharmacokinetic and pharmacodinamic parameters (table 1).

Table 1 PHARMACOKINETICS OF VARIOUS BENZODIAZEPINES

Drug	Peak time (hours)	Distribution volume (l/kg)	% Bound to plasma protein
Alprazolam	0.6-1.4	0.7-1.2	70
Bromazepam	0.5-8	0.86-1.56	70
Brotizolam	0.5-4	0.66	91
Chlordiazepoxide	1-2	0.33-0.41	94-97
Clobazam	1-4	0.87-2.83	83
Clonazepam	3-12	1.59	83-87
Clotiazepam	0.5-1.5	3.5	99
Diazepam	0.25-1.5	1.1	98-99
Flunitrazepam	1-1.5	2.2-4.1	80
Flurazepam	3	3.4	98
Loprazolam	0.5-4.5	2.83-31.5	80
Lorazepam	2	1.14-1.33	65-75
Midazolam	0.3-1	0.8-1.7	94-98
Nitrazepam	2	1.45-2.80	87
Oxazepam	1-5	0.2-2.3	87-96
Quazepam	2.4	5	97
Temazepam	0.3-1	1.3-1.6	96-98
Triazolam	0.7-2.5	1	89

The impact of pharmacokinetic factors on the clinical action has to be investigated in theoretical models, in which the pharmacodinamic variable must be considered as constant during the duration of the drug in the body. In the context of pharmacokinetic concept, two assumptions have been put forward:

i. plasma BDZs levels positively correlate with BDZs concentrations at the brain receptor sites

ii. clinical efficacy correlates with plasma concentrations above the minimal effective concentration, below which no clinical effects are contemplated.

Whereas the first notion is well accepted since BDZs are highly lipophilic and rapidly achieve equilibrium across the blood brain barrier, opinions differ about the second assumption. In fact, the concept of minimal effective concentration (Cmin) may change with the different clinical effects being examined and the methods used to quantify it.

After a single dose of BDZ, the onset of action depends largely on the absorption rate. The time to onset of clinical effect is the period from ingestion to the point at which Cmin is achieved — which is different from the time at which peak plasma concentrations are reached (Tmax). For example, with clonazepam the onset of clinical action occurs within 20-30 minutes, whereas peak plasma concentration is achieved between 1 and 2 hours after oral ingestion (McEvoy, 1989). Obviously, the higher the rate of absorption, the more Tpp approximates to, thus the absorption rate for a drug is a critical factor effecting the time required for the subjective effect to appear.

Those BDZs that are rapidly absorbed from the gastrointestinal tract have a prompt clinical action, whereas those that are slowly absorbed have a much slower onset of action. After oral administration, the absorption of diazepam, alprazolam, desmethyldiazepam (formed from its precursor clorazepate) fluorazepam (leading to its aldehyde and hydroxyethyl metabolites) midazolam and triazolam is very rapid (Weiershausen, 1985). Peak plasma concentration occurs about 1 hour after ingestion. Such rapid absorption accounts for the acute subjective high drowsiness, “spaced-out” feeling or motor impairment after the drug is ingested. Diazepam has a systemic bioavailability of 100%. Lorazepam, oxazepam and prazepam (which reaches the systemic circulation only in the form of active metabolites) are absorbed more slowly and achieve peak plasma concentration within 2 hours after oral administration. The bioavailability of oxazepam taken orally is about 60% (Greenblatt and Shader, 1987).

Rapid onset of action after oral dosage may represent a desirable objective for the treatment of sleep onset disorders. Conversely, for the treatment of anxiety, the benefits of a rapid onset of clinical efforts are much less defined. Whereas many subjects feel the prompt onset of action provided by rapidly absorbed BDZ is helpful, others experience the same effects as disturbing and unwanted. As a result, slowly and rapidly absorbed BDZs have to be prescribed according to the specific clinical situation as well as the sensitivity of the individual patient. All else being almost equal, BDZs absorption can be affected by several factors including food, concurrent therapy, formulation and subjects' position. Thus, a slowed and decreasing absorption occurs in the reclining position, in the presence of food in the stomach or if a BDZ is administered together with an aluminum containing antacid. Some tablets or hard gelatin capsules are absorbed less rapidly than the soft gelatin capsules containing BDZs in polyethylene glycol (McEvoy, 1989).

Irrespective of the routes of administration, plasma concentrations reached with BDZs show high interindividual variations. The intersubject variability is also observed for all other pharmacokinetic factors. After intramuscular injection of diazepam or chlordiazepoxide, absorption is slow (the plasma levels peaking at 10-12 hours) and erratic. As a consequence, clinical effects may be delayed and unpredictable (Greenblatt et al., 1983). The intramuscular route should be avoided for these drugs although lorazepam, clorazepam and midazolam are an exception, since they are well absorbed following i.m. injection. As the rates of intramuscular absorption of these drugs are superior to those obtained with an oral dose, the peak levels in the blood are higher and the clinical effect is greater (Shaefer, 1987).

Rectal administration of BDZs is rarely used considering the relatively low concentrations obtained with this route. An exception can be diazepam, which can achieve acceptable plasma levels when administered rectally in children.

No BDZs are available in a form for sublingual administration. Only lorazepam has been developed in this form — the idea being that bypassing the gastrointestinal tract would achieve minimal effective concentration more rapidly, while the time of onset of clinical effect would be similar to that obtained via the intramuscular route. However, no significant differences have been found between the absorption rates using either the sublingual or standard oral tablets (Greenblatt et al., 1982).

When BDZs are given by oral or intramuscular administration, the absorption rate from the gut or from the site of the injection appears to be the main step affecting the onset of clinical activity. Bypassing absorption through intravenous administration results in a more rapid onset of activity, mainly determined by the time taken for the drug to diffuse across the blood brain barrier. Therefore, the small variability in the time of onset of action exhibited by various BDZs following intravenous injection may be explained by differences in their lipid solubility (Greenblatt and Shader, 1985).

BDZ derivatives are extensively bound to serum proteins. The extent of binding varies considerably among drugs and ranges from about 70% for alprazolam to nearly 99% for diazepam. The primary binding protein for BDZs appears to be albumin, although triazolobenzodiazepines may bind to some degree to a acid glycoprotein. The binding decreases the concentration of free active drug in equilibrium with the sites of action and elimination, thereby reducing the intensity of action, but prolonging the effect and slowing the elimination (McKenzie, 1983). Table 1 shows the percentage of the bound fraction for the most common BDZs.

Glomerural filtration of many BDZs is low because of their extensive serum protein binding. Conversely, conditions of hypoalbuminemia occurring with age or with disease states including cirrhosis, renal insufficiency and severe burns results in higher levels of free active drug — and side effects such as drowsiness might be more frequent, since only unbound drug molecules have access to the central nervous system. The displacement of BDZ from the plasma binding site by another drug could modify its effect and possibly lead to drug interactions between this class and other pharmacological agents. However, very few clinically significant interactions involving BDZs appear to be based on competition for common binding sites on the plasma proteins (Greenblatt and Shader, 1985).

After peak plasma level is achieved, during the distribution phase, BDZs exhibit an initial rapid decline in plasma concentration, which then levels off into the more gradual decrease of the elimination phase. The curve representing variations of plasma concentrations over time shows a biphasic profile consistent with a two compartment model. In the initial phase (the alpha phase) the rate of decrement of plasma drug concentrations is the result of drug redistribution from the central (serum and brain) to peripheral compartments (including adipose tissue, skeletal muscle and liver). The extent of peripheral distribution (as determined by volume of distribution) increases as BDZs are more lipophilic. After distribution equilibrium is attained, the rate of drug disappearance from plasma enters a slower phase, the beta phase, which is indicative of drug elimination from the body, mainly by liver biotransformation and kidney clearance.

Hepatic metabolism accounts for the biotransformation of all BDZs. The two major pathways involved are microsomial oxidation, including N-dealkylation or aliphatic hydroxylation, and subsequent conjugation by glucuronic transfers to form glucuronides that are excreted in the urine. The pattern and rates of metabolism depend on the individual drugs (Hobbs et al., 1996).

For BDZs with a substituent group at position 1 or 2 of diazepine ring, the first step of metabolism involves the removal of the substituent with a formation of N-desalkylated biologically active compounds. Nordiazepam is the major metabolite common to the biotransformation of clorazepate, diazepam, halazepam and prazepam. It also derives from demoxepam (metabolite of chlordiazepoxide).

The subsequent step results in hydroxylation at position 3 which yields an active compound (e.g. oxazepam from nordiazepam). The conjugation of the 3-OH compounds with glucuronic acid represents the last stage.

Oxazepam, lorazepam and temazepam can be directly conjugated by virtue of their 3-OH group. The glucuronic conjugates are pharmacologically inactive and are excreted in the urine as such. The 7-nitro benzodiazepines, clonazepam and nitrazepam, are metabolized by the reduction of 7-nitro groups to form inactive amines, which are then acetylated before excretion. Alprazolam and triazolam are metabolized principally by initial hydroxylation of the methyl group on the fuse triazolo ring. Midazolam is rapidly metabolized, primarily by hydroxylation of the methyl group on the fused imidazolo ring.

Since BDZs do not seem to induce synthesis of hepatic microsomial enzymes, prolonged administration usually does not induce the accelerated metabolism of other drugs or of the BDZs. Oxidation, which results in active metabolites, is influenced by factors such as age, liver impairment, inhibition of liver enzymes by other drugs (cimetidine, oral contraceptives, isoniazid, phenytoin, propranolol, disulfiram). Conjugation is much less influenced by these factors, and therefore, theoretically at least, BDZs metabolized by conjugation are safer to use in the elderly or in patients with liver diseases. Renal insufficiency may impair excretion of glucuronide metabolites causing their accumulation, but this has not demonstrated pharmacologic consequences since the metabolites are inactive (Greenblatt et al., 1983).

Duration of Action

BDZs may be commonly classified according to pharmacokinetic parameters of half-life into three major groups:

a) Long acting BDZs such as diazepam, clobazam, clorazepate etc. In fact these display half-life values exceeding 24 hours, and in the process of liver biotransformation they generate long half-life active metabolites. Therefore, they accumulate extensively during repeated administration.
b) Intermediate and short acting BDZs, such as alprazolam, clonazepam, chlordiazepoxide, lorazepam, lormetezapam, oxazepam, nitrazepam and temazepam. Their half-life values range from 5 to 24 hours, and compounds metabolically generated are non active.
c) Ultra short acting BDZs, such as triazolam and midazolam. These have half-life values of less than 5 hours and are essentially non-accumulating.

The duration of pharmacological activity of BDZs does not correlate directly with the plasma concentration profiles of these drugs. For instance, the pharmacokinetic profile suggests that lorazepam, which has a more rapid half-life of elimination, would be a shorter acting BDZ than diazepam, if there was a direct correlation of effect with pharmacokinetics. However, lorazepam has been shown to have a longer duration pharmacological activity, suggesting that factors other than plasma half-life also have to be considered when assessing the duration of the pharmacological effects of BDZs (table 2).

Table 2 ELIMINATION HALF-LIFE OF THE MOST USED BENZODIAZEPINES

Compound	Half-life (hours)
Prazepam	1.24
Flurazepam	1.60-5.30
Clorazepate	1.65-2.66
Midazolam	1.98
Ketazolam	2.00
Triazolam	2.9
Brotizolam	5.37
Oxazepam	6.18
Loprazolam	6.30
Clotiazepam	6.50-17.00
Alprazolam	11.01
Temazepam	12.35
Chlordiazepoxide	12.62-23.26
Lorazepam	12.90
Flunitrazepam	14.97-25.43
Nitrazepam	26.50
Quazepam	30.97
Clonazepam	32.37
Desmethyldiazepam (clorazepate)	42.67
Diazepam	54.00

Values were obtained from Woods et al., (1992)

BDZs have to cross the blood-brain barrier (BBB) to achieve their pharmacological effects. The physiochemical properties which influence the rate and extent of drug entry into cerebrospinal fluid (CSF)/brain are protein binding, lipid solubility and pKa ionization constant. Drug molecules which are lipophylic, non-ionized and not bound to proteins may readily cross BBB and a rapid distribution may be achieved between blood, CSF and brain (Colburn and Jack, 1987). More precisely, the entry into CSF/brain (and hence the onset of pharmacological activity of BDZs) is dependent on their lipophilicity. The more lipophilic the compound, the more rapid the onset of clinical activity. Therefore, the amount of BDZ available to enter the CSF/brain compartment is limited by protein binding, since only the free fraction of the total BDZ-blood concentration can cross BBB. Both animal and human investigations with diazepam, chlordiazepoxide and desmethyldiazepam have shown that CSF concentrations are equivalent to the free drug concentrations in the blood, confirming that protein binding regulates the amount of drug available to cross BBB (Halstrom et al., 1980; Stanski et al., 1976).

The affinity for binding to the BDZ receptor influences both the pharmacological potency and the duration of activity of these compounds. The magnitude of the clinical doses are directly proportional to the inhibition constant (Ki). Lorazepam and nitrazepam have a greater affinity for the receptor than diazepam and chlordiazepoxide (Speth et al., 1978). The elimination half-life of nitrazepam, for example, is 27 and 68 hours in the blood and in CSF respectively, whereas compounds such as diazepam and chlordiazepoxide exhibit the same elimination half-life in both blood and CSF (Stanski et al., 1976; Kangas et al., 1977; Greenblatt et al., 1980). Consequently, nitrazepam and lorazepam, with a greater affinity for receptor binding sites, exhibit apparently longer elimination half-lives in CSF than in plasma, and prolonged clinical effects. The release of nitrazepam and lorazepam from the receptor sites would thus become the rate-limiting step in drug clearance from the body, rather than metabolism per se. In other words, diazepam and chlordiazepoxide plasma levels may be more predictive of the duration of pharmacological activity because they parallel the CSF concentration of these drugs. Conversely, the slower CSF elimination half-lives and the longer duration of pharmacological activity of lorazepam and nitrazepam are not predictable from plasma concentration, but are predictable from the high affinity of these compounds for the brain receptor sites (Colburn and Jack, 1987).

Since plasma free drug concentrations are similar to the CSF drug concentrations available for receptor binding, the free drug concentrations-time profile, along with the association and dissociation rate constants for the receptor, can be used to establish the time course of receptor occupancy, and the clinical effect profile. At this point, the relative contribution of active compounds metabolically generated to the actual duration of the pharmacological action of BDZs has to be evaluated in order to identify further factors determining duration of activity of BDZ medications.

In fact, as reported above, many BDZs are biotransformed into pharmacologically active metabolites, which in turn appear in the systemic circulation in an unconjugated and therefore potentially important clinical form. This prompts the recognition of which metabolites participate in clinical activity, and the relative tribute of each metabolite to the activity of the parent compound. The assessment of the clinical importance of endogenously formed metabolites thus involves the simultaneous consideration of several aspects including:
a) the quantitative extent to which a specific metabolite is formed
b) the extent to which it reaches the brain receptor sites
c) the affinity of the individual metabolite for the central receptor sites.

The following examples may be helpful in understanding this issue. For instance, during prolonged treatment with diazepam plasma levels of its metabolite desmethyldiazepam equal or exceed those of parent. Desmethyldiazepam lipophilicity is similar to that of diazepam — the brain/free blood concentration ratios for the two drugs are almost the same (Guentert, 1984). In addition, the active metabolite has a higher affinity for the binding site (Miller et al., 1987). Taken together, these data suggest that desmethyldiazepam is an important participant in the clinical activity of diazepam during chronic therapy. On the other hand, during chronic treatment with clobazam its metabolite desmethylclobazam yields plasma concentrations exceeding those of the parent drug by at least twofold (Klotz et al., 1980; Ochs et al., 1984). The brain/free plasma level ratios between the two compounds are similar. However, since the binding affinity of desmethylclobazam is more than ten times inferior to that of clobazam, it is unlikely that the metabolite can participate in the clinical action of clobazam (Miller et al., 1987). The active metabolite desalkyflurazepam of both flurazepam and quazepam has about a sixfold higher affinity for benzodizepine binding sites than either parent compound — whereas for alprazolam, midazolam and triazolam, their metabolites show a lower affinity for the binding sites than the parent compounds (Ankier and Goa, 1988; Arendt et al., 1987).

Knowledge of both the receptor binding affinities and pharmacokinetic properties of BDZs may therefore be helpful in determining the rational clinical use of these drugs. This will be especially important during chronic medication with molecules that have active metabolites with a higher affinity for BDZ binding sites than the parent compound.

Bibliography

Ankier SI and Goa KL: Quazepam: a preliminary review of its pharmacodynamic and pharmacokinetic properties, and therapeutic efficacy in insomnia. *Drugs* 35:42-62, 1988

Arendt RM, Greenblatt DJ, Liebisch DC, Luu MD and Paul SM: Determinants of benzodiazepine brain uptake: lipophilicity versus binding affinity. *Psychopharmacology* 93:72-76, 1987

Colburn WA and Jack ML: Relationship between CSF drug concentrations, receptor binding characteristics, and pharmacokinetic and pharmacodynamic properties of selected 1,4-substituted benzodiazepines. *Clinical Pharmacokinetics* 13:179-190, 1987

Greenblatt DJ, Divoll M, Abernethy DR, et al.: Benzodiazepine kinetics: implications for therapeutics and pharmacogeriatrics. *Drug Metabolism Reviews* 14:251-292, 1983

Greenblatt DJ, Divoll M, Harmatz JJ, et al.: Pharmacokinetic comparison of sublingual lorazepam with intravenous, intramuscular and oral lorazepam. *Journal of Pharmaceutical Sciences* 71:248-252, 1982

Greenblatt DJ, Ochs HR, Lloyd BL.: Entry of diazepam and its major metabolite into cerebrospinal fluid. *Psychopharmacology* 70:89-93, 1980

Greenblatt DJ and Shader RI: Clinical pharmacokinetics of the benzodiazepines. In Smith DE, Wesson DR, eds. *The benzodiazepines: current standards for medical practice*. Lancaster, MTP Press, 1985

Greenblatt DJ and Shader RI: The pharmacokinetics of anti-anxiety agents. In: Meltzer HY, ed. *Psychopharmacology: the third generation of progress*. Raven Press, New York 1987

Greenblatt DJ, Shader RI and Abernethy DR: Current status of benzodiazepines (first of two parts). *New England Journal Medicine* 309:354-358, 1983

Guentert TW: Pharmacokinetics of benzodiazepines and of their metabolites. In: *Progress in Drug Metabolism*. Bridges, JG and Chasseaud LF (eds.). Taylor and Francis, London 8:241-386, 1984

Halstrom C, Lader MH and Curry SH: Diazepam and desmethyldiazepam concentrations in saliva, plasma and CSF. *British Journal of Clinical Pharmacology* 9:333-339, 1980

Hobbs WR, Rall TW and Verdoorn TA: Hypnotics and sedatives; ethanol. In: *Goodman and Gilman's the pharmacological basis of therapeutics*. Hardman JG, Limbird LE, Molinoff PB, Ruddon RW and Goodman Gilman A (eds.). 9th Edition McGraw-Hill, New York pp. 361-396, 1996

Kangas L, Kanto J., Siirtola T and Pekkarinen A: Cerebrospinal fluid concentrations of nitrazepam in man. *Acta Pharmacologica et Toxicologica* 41:74-79, 1977

Kaplan SA, Jack ML, Alexander K and Weinfeld RE: Pharmacokinetic profile of diazepam in man following single intravenous and oral and chronic oral administrations. *Journal of Pharmaceutical Sciences* 62:1789-1796, 1973.

Klotz U, Kargas L and Kanto J: Clinical pharmacokinetcs of benzodiazepines. *Progress Pharmacol* 3(No. 3):1-72, 1980

McEvoy GK (ed.) *American Hospital Formulary Service Drug Information*. Bethesda MD: American Society of Hospital Pharmacists, Inc., 1989

McKenzie SG: Introduction to the pharmacokinetics and pharmacodynamics of benzodiazepines. *Progress in Neuropsychopharmacology and Biological Psychiatry* 7:623-627, 1983

Miller LG, Greenblatt DJ, Paul SM and Shader RI: Benzodiazepine receptor occupancy in vivo: correlation with brain concentrations and pharmacodynamic ac-

tions. *Journal of Pharmacology and Experimental Therapeutics* 240:516-522, 1987
Miller LG, Greenblatt DJ and Shader RI: Benzodiazepine receptor binding: influence of physiologic and pharmacologic factors. *Biopharm Drug Disposition* 8:103-114, 1987
Ochs HR, Greenblatt DJ, Luttkenhorst M and Verburg-Ochs B: Single and multiple dose kinetics of clobazam, and clinical effects during multiple dosage. *European Journal of Clinical Pharmacology* 26:499-503, 1984
Shaefer MS: The newer benzodiazepines lorazepam and midazolam. *Seminars in Interventional Radiology* 4:173-178, 1987
Stanski DR, Greenblatt DJ, Selwyn A Shader RI, Franke K, et al.: Plasma and cerebrospinal fluid concentrations of chlordiazepoxide and its metabolites in surgical patients. *Clinical Pharmacology and Therapeutics* 20:571-578, 1976
Speth RC, Wastek GJ, Johnson PC and Yamamura HI: Benzodiazepine binding in human brain: characterization using [^{3}H] flunitrazepam. *Life Sciences* 22:859-866, 1978
Weiershausen U: Pharmacokinetic considerations in the treatment of chronic anxiety. In: Smith DE and Wesson DR (eds.) *The benzodiazepines: current standards for medical practice*. Lancaster, MTP Press, 1985
Woods J H, Katz J L and Winger G: Benzodiazepines: use, abuse, and consequences. *Pharmacological Reviews* 44:151-347, 1992

Alprazolam

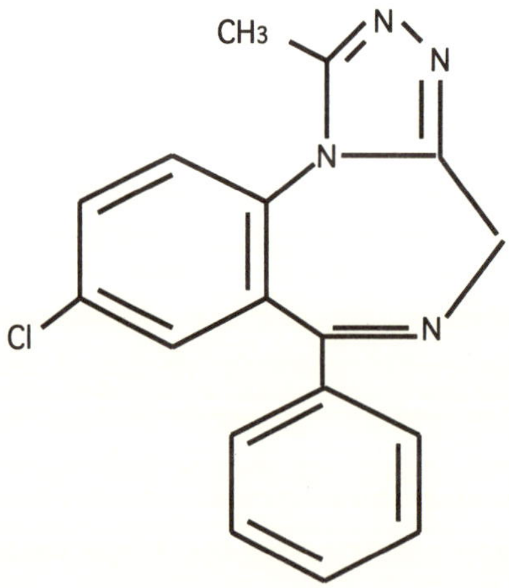

CH3 N N N Cl N

ALPRAZOLAM

Alprazolam is the first of the class of compounds referred to as the 1,4 triazolo-benzodiazepine. As such, it has the 1,4 triazolo ring, a 5 membered heterocycle, fused on position 1,2 of the BDZ nucleus.

Absorption of alprazolam is characteristically rapid, with peak concentrations occurring within 1 hour after administration. Following a single dose of

0.028 mg/Kg, mean peak plasma concentration of 40 μg/l is reached in 1.3 hours. Average steady-state concentrations obtained in subjects receiving multiple oral doses of 1 mg (3, 6 and 9 mg/die) are 29.3, 61.5 and 102.9 μg/l respectively. Thus, alprazolam appears to exhibit linear pharmacokinetics over the dosage ranges used. Although alprazolam absorption is slower when the drug is co-administered with meals, the difference in Tmax is not significant. The absorption half-lives seem to be significantly longer in young women than in elderly women (31.9 versus 13.1 minutes) with peak serum levels lower (15.7 versus 25.9 μg/l). But Cmax and Tmax values do not show any significant difference between young and elderly men (Ciraulo et al., 1986; Ellinwood et al., 1985; Scavone et al., 1987). Systemic bioavailability is estimated to be more than the 92% after oral administration (Smith et al., 1984). The distribution volume of alprazolam is approximately 0.8 l/Kg after 1 mg oral tablet. It appears to be greater in young men (1.17 l/Kg) than in elderly men (0.9 l/Kg) whereas age does not affect this parameter in women (Eberts et al., 1980). Alprazolam is 68.4% bound to plasma proteins and the extent of binding is independent of drug concentrations over a range from 10 to 10,000 μg/l (Moschitto and Greenblatt, 1983).

The 1,4 triazolo ring prevents the oxidative metabolism of the classical BDZs, which results in the generation of active metabolites with long elimination half-lives. Alprazolam is largely metabolized. It undergoes hydroxylation induced by microsomial enzymes in the liver. The major product is α-hydroxyalprazolam, which accounts for 17% of the total amounts recovered in the urine. Although it displays central pharmacological activity as suggested by binding assay (Ki=4.2 nM) (Sethy and Harris, 1982), it is unlikely that α-hydroxy derivative is involved in alprazolam's in vivo effects, since its plasma concentration never exceeds 10% of the levels of the unchanged parent drug (Smith and Kroboth, 1987). Other metabolites identified in the urine in negligible amounts are 4-hydroxy-alprazolam, α-4-hydroxy-alprazolam and 3-methyl-triazolyl. They account for 0.3%, 0.2% and 0.9% respectively (Eberts et al., 1980).

The mean elimination half-life of alprazolam ranges from 9.5 to 12 hours. Its major metabolite α-hydroxy-alprazolam shows a shorter elimination half-life of 1-2 hours (Smith and Kroboth, 1987). Liver disease prolongs alprazolam elimination, whereas renal dysfunction does not. Therefore, alprazolam accumulation would not occur in subjects suffering from kidney insufficiency — but dosage adjustments would be required in situations of liver illness, based on alterations in pharmacokinetics. Sex differences do not appear to significantly influence the pharmacokinetic parameters of alprazolam during multiple dose administration. But alprazolam elimination half-life is prolonged in obese compared to control subjects (Abernethy et al., 1984).

The reported drug-drug interaction represents predominantly the effect of the inhibition of the microsomial enzyme system responsible for the hepatic metabolism and elimination of alprazolam. For example, concomitant administration of cimetidine with multiple doses of alprazolam would result in elevated steady state plasma alprazolam concentrations. A reduced daily dosage of alprazolam or an increased dosing interval is therefore suggested if the two drugs are coadministered. In the same way, since the influence of low estrogen oral contraceptives on the pharmacokinetics of alprazolam involves a prolonged elimination half-life, a lower daily dose of alprazolam is advisable in women using contraceptives.

Bibliography

Abernethy DR, Greenblatt DJ, Divoll M, Smith RB and Shader RI: The influence of obesity on the pharmacokinetics of oral alprazolam and triazolam. *Clinical Pharmacokinetics* 9:177-183, 1984

Ciraulo DA, Barnhill JG, Boxebaum HG, Greenblatt DJ and Smith RB: Pharmacokinetics and clinical effects of alprazolam following single and multiple oral doses in patients with panic disorder. *Journal of Clinical Pharmacology* 26:292-298, 1986

Eberts FS, Pilopoulos Y, Reineke LM and Vliek RW: Disposition of ^{14}C-alprazolam, a new anxiolytic antidepressant in man. *Abstract Pharmacologist* 22:279, 1980

Ellinwood EH, Heatherly DG, Nikardo AM, Bjornsson TD and Kilts C: Comparative pharmacokinetics and pharmacodynamics of lorazepam, alprazolam and diazepam. *Psychopharmacology* 86:392-399, 1985

Moschitto LJ and Greenblatt DJ: Concentration-independent plasma protein binding of benzodiazepines. *Journal of Pharmacy and Pharmacology* 35:179-180, 1983

Scavone JM, Greenblatt DJ and Shader RI: Alprazolam kinetics following sublingual and oral administration. *Journal of Clinical Psychopharmacology* 7:332-334, 1987

Sethy VH and Harris DW: Determination of biological activity of alprazolam, triazolam and their metabolites. *Journal of Pharmacy and Pharmacology* 34:115-116, 1982

Smith RB and Kroboth PD: Influence of dosing regimen on alprazolam and metabolite serum concentration and tolerance to sedative and psychomotor effects. *Psychopharmacology* 93:105-112, 1987

Smith RB, Kroboth PD, Vanderlugt JT, Phillips JP and Juhl RP: Pharmacokinetics and pharmacodynamics of alprazolam after oral and IV administration. *Psychopharmacology* 84:452-456, 1984

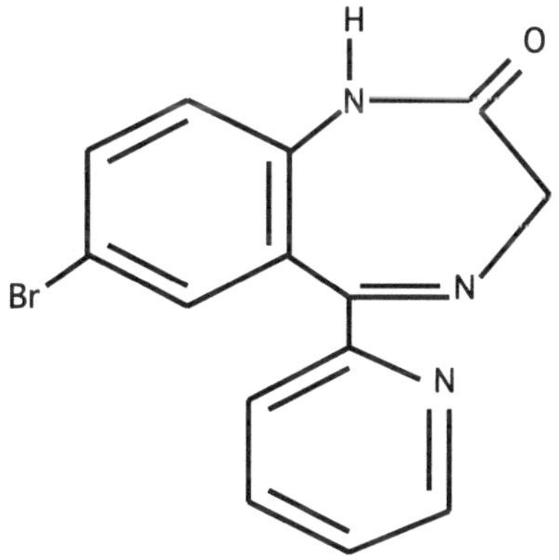

Bromazepam

Bromazepam is rapidly absorbed after oral administration. Following a single dose of 6 mg, peak serum concentrations are reached in 1-2 hours from administration and range from 60 to 80 µg/l. A longer absorption time is required when bromazepam is administered in tablet form. Following the oral administration of 12 mg of bromazepam as a tablet, blood level maxima occur between 1 and 4 hours, and the blood level peaks range from 107 to 173 µg/l (Guentert, 1984; Clausen et al., 1989).

It has been reported that after a single oral bromazepam administration, blood level plateaux in most subjects are observed subsequent to a relatively rapid onset of peak concentrations. This could be explained by the intrinsic dissolution characteristics of bromazepam at various pH values: moderate dissolution rate and reduced extend of solubility at higher pH (Kaplan et al., 1976). This means that if the drug is not completely dissolved in the strongly acidic environment of the stomach, prolonged intestinal absorption at a slow rate can occur.

When bromazepam is coadministered with meals, the rate of absorption is slower. The peak concentration and AUC value of bromazepam are significantly lower under a non-fasting condition than in a fasting situation (Fujii et al., 1990). No differences concerning the elimination processes of bromazepam have been observed between the two conditions. Food ingestion can influence tablet disintegration, drug dissolution, gastrointestinal secretion, and the rate of gastric emptying. These mechanisms are probably responsible for the food-induced alteration bromazepam's bioavailability.

Compared to other benzodiazepines, the disposition kinetics of bromazepam is relatively simple. After intravenous administration, the plasma drug concentration-time course is, in most cases, sufficiently described using a one-compartment model. An apparent volume distribution of between 50% and 90% of body weight and a total body clearance close to 0.5 ml/min/Kg have been reported (Raaflaub and Speiser-Courvoisier, 1974). According to different studies, the half-lives range from 15 to 20 hours (Guentert, 1984; Kaplan et al., 1976; Raaflaub and Speiser-Courvoisier, 1974; von Stetten et al., 1983; Ascalone et al., 1984). A more recent study is the only one to observe half-life values slightly higher than those previously reported, 20 hours in young healthy male and 29 hours in female (Ochs et al., 1987). Although bromazepam has previously been considered to be a "short" or "intermediate" half-life benzodiazepine, its half-life value falls in the "intermediate to long" range.

After administration of 6 or 12 mg of bromazepam, a mean 70% of the dose is recovered in the urine, but only 2.3% of the dose is excreted unchanged in the urine (Raaflaub and Speiser-Courvoisier, 1974; Kaplan et al., 1976).

Bromazepam in plasma is 70% bound to proteins (Raaflaub and Speiser-Courvoisier, 1974). Compared to other benzodiazepines, bromazepam free fraction is relatively high. In contrast to some other BDZs, no metabolites of bromazepam have been identified with a longer elimination half-life than the parent compound.

The overall elimination rate constant and the half-life of elimination of bromazepam on day 30 of chronic administration are essentially the same of those reported following a single dose administration of bromazepam (Kaplan et al., 1976).

The presence of a pyridil ring substituent in the 5-position of the benzodiazepine molecule induces a marked decrease in the lipophilicity of the molecule and a faster hydroxylation in position 3, when compared to other benzodiazepines in the same group.

The major metabolic pathway of bromazepam in humans involves hepatic oxidative biotransformation, yielding 3-hydroxybromazepam as the the major metabolite (Kaplan et al., 1976; Sawada and Hara, 1978). The 3-hydroxybromazepam, a pharmacologically active metabolite, is so rapidly conjugated and excreted that bromazepam itself is probably responsible for essential pharmacological activity. Aromatic ring hydroxylation yields 9- and 5'-hydroxybromazepam in various species.

Cleavage of the diazepine ring of bromazepam leads to the formation of 2-(2-amino-5-bromobenzoil) pyridine and 2-(2-amino-5-bromo-3-hydroxybenzoil)pyridine. This last compound is the major metabolite in humans, rabbits, and dogs (Sawada and Hara, 1978).

Bromazepam clearance is significantly impaired in elderly persons, aged

60 to 81 years, compared to those of both sexes aged between 21 and 31 years. (Ochs et al., 1987). The average reduction is nearly 50%. This indicates that the steady-state concentration of bromazepam at any given dosing rate would be nearly twice as high in an elderly, compared to a young patient. Peak serum bromazepam concentrations after oral doses of bromazepam are also significantly higher in elderly subjects. This is not because of a different rate of absorption because the time of peak serum bromazepam concentration is not influenced by age. It is probably due to a well known reduction in lean body mass in the elderly, with a concurrent increase in adipose tissue relative to total body weight. Bromazepam is a relatively nonlipophilic benzodiazepine, and the reduced volume of distribution with age probably reflects reduced peripheral distribution in the elderly. These data may indicate that older persons would be more sensitive to the clinical action of bromazepam (Ochs et al., 1987).

No significant differences in bromazepam clearance have been observed between contraceptive and noncontraceptive female users (Ochs et al., 1987).

Coadministration of bromazepam with therapeutic doses of cimetidine leads to a significant 50% reduction in total clearance of bromazepam, with a significant prolongation of half-life elimination. Coadministration of these two drugs could consequently lead to increased steady-state serum bromazepam concentrations, with the accompanying probability of increased clinical effects (Ochs et al., 1987).

Propranolol coadministration with bromazepam also induces a reduction of bromazepam clearance and an enhancement of elimination half-life by an average of 20%. The half-life prolongation is statistically significant — the reduction in clearance is not (Ochs et al., 1987).

Bibliography

Ascalone V, Cisternino M, Sicolo N and DePalo E: Bioavailability of bromazepam in man after single administration of an oral solution. *Arzneimittelforschung* 34:96-98, 1984

Clausen TG, Boysen K and Larsen F: Plasma concentrations of bromazepam following peroral and sublingual administration. *Pharmacology and Toxicology* 64:389-390, 1989

Fujii J, Inotsume N and Nakano M: Effect of food on the bioavailability of bromazepam following oral administration in healthy volunteers. *Journal Pharmacobio Dyn* 13:269-271, 1990

Guentert TW: Pharmacokinetics of benzodiazepines and of their metabolites. In: *Progress in drug metabolism*, Bridges JW and Chasseaud LF (eds) Taylor and Francis Ltd., London UK and Philadelphia PA, Vol 8, pp. 241-386, 1984

Kaplan SA, Jack ML, Weinfeld RE, Glover W, Weissman L and Cotler S: Biopharmaceutical and clinical pharmacokinetic profile of bromazepam. *Journal of Pharmacokinetics and Biopharmaceut* 4:1-16, 1976

Ochs HR, Greenblatt DJ, Friedman H, Burstein ES, Locniskar A, Harmatz JS and Shader RI: Bromazepam pharmacokinetics: influence of age, gender, oral contraceptives, cimetidine, and propranolol. *Clinical Pharmacology and Therapeutics* 41:562-570, 1987

Raaflaub VJ and Speiser-Courvoisier J: On the pharmacokinetics of bromazepam in man. *Arzneimittelforschung* 24:1841-1844, 1974

Sawada H and Hara A: Studies on metabolism of bromazepam. VI Reduction of 2-(2-amino-5bromobenzoyl)pyridine, a metabolite of bromazepam, in rabbit, rat, and guinea pig. *Drug Metabolism and Disposition* 6:205-212, 1978

von Stetten VO, Rehm KD, Fenzl E, Barkworth MF and Johnson KI: Comparative studies on the bioavailability and pharmacokinetics of bromazepam from tablets. *Arzneimittelforschung* 33:1699-1702, 1983

Brotizolam

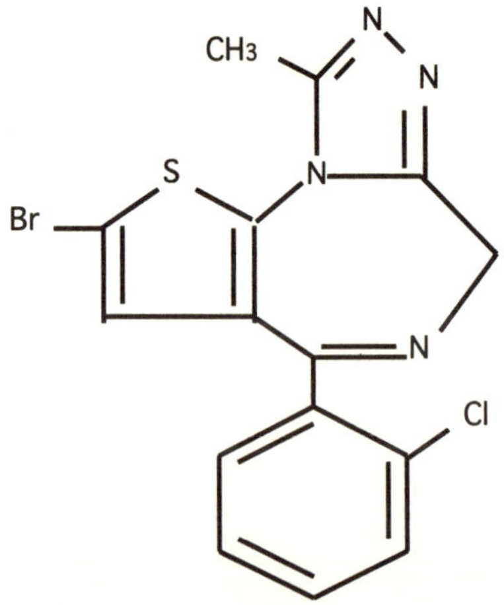

CH3 N N N S Br N Cl

BROTIZOLAM

Brotizolam is a thienotiazolo substituted diazepine derivative which possesses pharmacological properties characteristic of the BDZ class of drugs. Brotizolam is well absorbed from the gastrointestinal tract. Following single oral doses of 0.25 to 1 mg brotizolam, peak plasma levels are observed within 2 hours (0.5-4 hours) (Bechtel, 1983). There appears to be a linear correlation between dose and mean maximum plasma concentration over a range dose up to 1.5 mg, since at higher doses the increase in Cmax is markedly blunted (Bechtel, 1984). Its bioavailability, estimated after an oral dose of 0.5 mg, averages 70% (Jochemsen et al., 1983).

Brotizolam distributes rapidly through the body. Following intravenous injection of 0.25 mg, plasma concentrations decline according to an open-two compartment model. The mean half-life of the distribution or alpha phase is 11 minutes, with intersubject variations ranging from 4.3 to 19.8 minutes (Jochemsen et al., 1983). After an oral dose of 0.25 mg of brotizolam, the distribution half-life ranges between 7 and 26 minutes. The mean apparent distribution volume is 0.66 l/Kg calculated after 0.25 mg of brotizolam was injected intravenously to healthy volunteers (Bechtel et al., 1986b).

Animal studies show that brotizolam easily passes into breast milk and crosses the placenta (Bechtel et al., 1986a). By using an equilibrium dialysis technique, brotizolam appears to be extensively bound to plasma proteins with only 8.4% remaining free (Jochemsen et al., 1983c, 1983d). In people, brotizolam is rapidly and almost completely metabolized in the liver. Hydroxylation at different sites produces 1-metylhydroxy and 4-hydroxy-brotizolam that represent the main metabolites. They possess some pharmacological activity but are less potent that the parent drug (Danneberg et al., 1986). They are further catabolized to inactive conjugates of glucuronic or sulphuric acid and excreted in the urine. Less then 1% of the administered dose of brotizolam is eliminated via the kidney as unchanged drug. Excretion of a single dose is terminated within 4 days. Mean elimination half-life averages between 3.5 and 7.8 hours and is usually about 5 hours. Short elimination half-life is prolonged in the elderly with mean values up to 9.7 hours (Jochemsen et al., 1983b). Kidney insufficiency does not significantly influence brotizolam elimination which, in fact is increased in subjects with liver diseases (Jochemsen et al., 1983a). A number of investigations demonstrate that neither brotizolam nor its derivatives accumulate with repeated administration (Greenblatt et al., 1983).

Bibliography

Bechtel WD: Pharmacokinetics and metabolism of brotizolam in humans. *British Journal of Clinical Pharmacology* 16:279S-283S, 1983

Bechtel WD: Radioreceptor assay of brotizolam in human plasma. *Fresenins Zeitschrift fur Analytische Chemie* 317:714-715, 1984

Bechtel WD, Mierau J, Brandt K, Forster HJ and Pook KH: Metabolic fate of ^{14}C-brotizolam in the rat, dog, monkey and man. *Arzneimittel-Forschung* 36:578-586, 1986a

Bechtel WD, van Weyjen RGA and van den Ende A: Blood level, excretion and metabolism pattern of ^{14}C-brotizolam in humans. *Arzneimittel-Forschung* 36:575-578, 1986b

Danneberg P, Boke-Kuhu, Bechtel WD and Lehr E: Pharmacological action of some known and possible metabolites of brotizolam. *Arzneimittel-Forschung* 36:587-591, 1986

Greenblatt DJ, Locniskar A, Shader RI and Pilot: pharmacokinetic study of brotizolam, a thienodiazepine hypnotic, using electron-capture gas-liquid chromatography. *Sleep* 6:72-76, 1983
Jochemsen R, Jores RP, Wesselman JGJ, Richter E and Breimer DD: Pharmacokinetics of oral brotizolam in patients with liver cirrhosis. *British Journal of Clinical Pharmacology* 16: 315S-322S, 1983a
Jochemsen R, Naudi KL, Corless D, Wesselman JGJ and Breimer DD: Pharmacokinetics of brotizolam in the elderly. *British Journal of Clinical Pharmacology* 16:299S-307S, 1983b
Jochemsen R, Wesselman JGJ, Hermans J, van Boxtel CJ and Breimer DD: Pharmacokinetics of brotizolam in healty subjects following intravenous and oral administration. *British Journal of Clinical Pharmacology* 16:285S-290S, 1983c
Jochemsen R, Wesselman JGJ, van Boxtel CJ, Hermans J and Breimer DD: Comparative pharmacokinetics of brotizolam and triazolam in healthy subjects. *British Journal of Clinical Pharmacology* 16:291S-297S, 1983d

Chlordiazepoxide

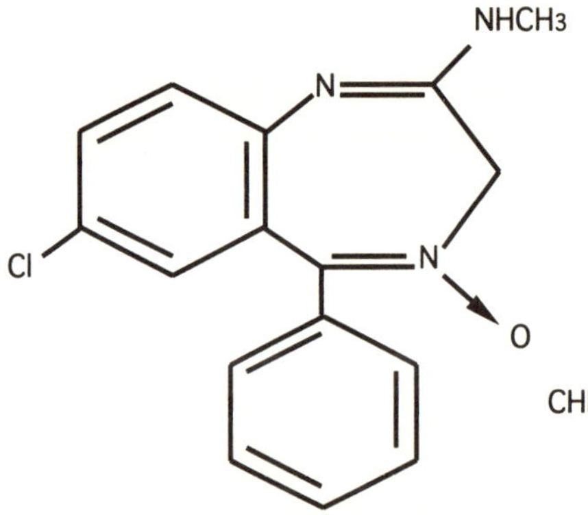

NHCH3
N
Cl
N
O
CHLORDIAZEPOXIDE

After oral administration chlordiazepoxide is completely absorbed with nearly 100% systemic bioavailability. Peak plasma concentrations are reached in 1-2 hours (Greenblatt et al., 1978). It is poorly absorbed through intramuscular injection and peak plasma levels are seen after 6-7 hours. Since this route results in a slow and incomplete absorption, and is painful (because of acidity of the solvent solution, the pH is adjusted upwards to pH 3), intramuscular injection should be prescribed only to patients who are vomiting or unable to take oral medication.

Chlordiazepoxide is 94% bound to serum albumin (Muller and Wollert, 1973). It is largely distributed throughout the body by virtue of its high lipid solubility with an apparent distribution volume of 0.33-0.41 l/Kg (Morselli et al., 1973). The highest concentrations are detected in the brain and adipose tissue, while CSF levels parallel the unbound plasma concentrations (Hallstrom et al., 1980).

Chlordiazepoxide passes into milk — 10% of the circulating amount has been found in the breast milk of lactating women taking the drug in a multiple dose schedule (Cree et al., 1973). It has also been measured in the umbilical blood in concentrations similar to those found in the mother. Therefore, because a new born has an impaired drug catabolism, levels of chlordiazepoxide as high as those of the mother provoke a weakness and hypotonia in the infant (Klotz, 1983).

The mean plasma half-life of chlordiazepoxide is about 15 hours with a range of 5.30 hours. It is widely metabolized with very little unchanged drug excreted.

There are two major pathways of hepatic catabolism:

a) the first pass involves a N-desmethylation which forms an active metabolite desmethyl-chlordiazepoxide with a mean half-life of 45 hours and desmethyldiazepam with an half-life of approximately 50 hours. Oxazepam is the last derivative produced along this route.
b) the second pathway involves hydrolysis of demoxepam to an open lactam.

Both glucuronic acid conjugates deriving from oxazepam and water soluble lactam are inactive derivatives which are excreted via urine and faeces. More than ten metabolites of chlorazepoxide have been identified: only three — desmethyl chlordiazepoxide, demozepam and desmethyldiazepam— possess biological activity. Since they display long half-lives and accumulate in the body during chronic treatment, they have an important involvement in determining the pharmacological activity of the parent drug (Boston Collaborative Drug Surveillance Program, 1973).

Bibliography

Boston Collaborative Drug Surveillance Program: Clinical depression in the CNS due to diazepam and chlordiazepoxide in relation to cigarette smoking and age. *New England Journal of Medicine*, 1973

Cree J, Meyer J and Hailey D: Diazepam in labour: its metabolism and effect on clinical conditions and thermogenesis of the newborn. *British Medical Journal* 4:251-255, 1973

Greenblatt DJ, Shader R, Franke K and Harmatz J: Pharmacokinetics of chlordiazepoxide and metabolites following single and multiple oral doses. *International Journal of Clinical Pharmacology and Biopharmaceutics* 16:486-493, 1978

Hallstrom C, Lader M and Curry S: Diazepam and N-desmethyldiazepam concentration in saliva, plasma and CSF. *British Journal of Clinical Pharmacology* 9:333-339, 1980

Klotz U: Clinical pharmacokinetics of benzodiazepines. In: *The Benzodiazepines: from Molecular Biology to Clinical Practice*. Costa E (ed.) Raven Press, New York, pp. 247-252, 1983

Morselli P, Cassano G, Placidi G, Muscettola G and Rizzo: Kinetics of the distribution of ^{14}C-diazepam and its metabolites in various areas of the cat brain. In: *The Benzodiazepines*. Garattini S, Mussini E and Randall L (eds.) Raven Press, New York, pp. 129-144, 1973

Muller W and Wollert U: Characterization of the binding of benzodiazepines to human serum albumin. *Naunyn-Schmiedeberg's Archives of Pharmacology* 280:229-237, 1973

Clobazam

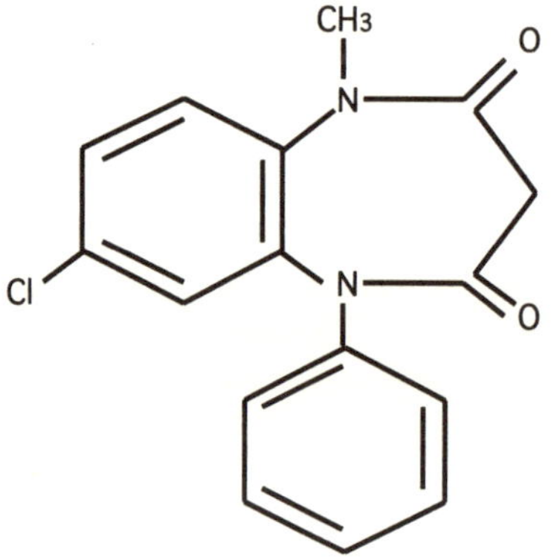

CH3
O
N
Cl
N
O

CLOBAZAM

Clobazam differs from the classic 1,4 benzodiazepine, e.g. diazepam, in that two nitrogens atoms are at positions 1 and 5 of the diazepine ring. Moreover, a keto group is located at position 4. Clobazam is the only one of the 1.5 benzodiazepines used in human therapy at present.

After oral administration, it is rapidly and almost completely absorbed (more than 87%). Peak serum concentrations are reached between 1 and 4 hours after administration, irrespective of the dose. 40 mg of clobazam yields peak serum levels ranging from 450 to 600 μg/l (Rupp et al., 1979). When clobazam is coadministered with meals, the rate of absorption is slowed, but neither the completeness of absorption nor the elimination-rate are affected (Divoll et al., 1982). Chemically, clobazam behaves as a neutral substance, and its absorption is not modified by the changes in the gastrointestinal tract. Its bioavailability does not differ if administered as a tablet or in solutions (Vallner et al., 1978).

Clobazam in the blood is carried extensively bound to proteins with a free fraction of approximately 16.9% (Volz et al., 1979). It is rapidly distributed to tissues, because of its high lipophilicity. Brain concentrations for both clobazam and its main metabolite, desmethyl-clobazam, are similar to those unbound in the plasma. The affinity for the brain receptor site displayed by desmethyl-clobazam is ten times less than that of clobazam (Arendt et al., 1987). Clobazam passes into the breast-milk: in women under prolonged medication more than 25% of the amounts measured in the blood may be detected in the milk.

The curve showing clobazam plasma concentrations over time has a classic bimodel profile:

- the alpha phase, rapid, with an half-life of 2.3 hours approximately
- then a slower elimination phase with an half-life in the range of 2.7 to 5.9 days.

This long half-life may be explained by the occurrence of metabolic products with a much slower termination half-life than the parent drug. In fact, N-desmethyl-clobazam has an elimination half-life of more than 40 hours, almost twice that of clobazam (Rupp et al., 1979).

Clobazam elimination is also affected by age since a minor clearance and a prolonged half-life have been found in the elderly (Greenblatt et al., 1981). The drug is metabolized in the liver. The main pathways involve first a dealkilation process yielding desmethyl-clobazam, which undergoes an hydroxylation at the position 4 of the aromatic group. Introduction of the hydroxy function at the 4 position of the phenyl ring without any previous dealkylation process represents a minor pathway which results in the production of the 4-hydroxy-clobazam.

All metabolites with an hydroxyl group on the aromatic ring are inactivated by conjugation with glucuronic acid (or sulphoric acid). Investigations in humans using labelled clobazam show that the main plasma metabolite is N-desmethyl-clobazam (M9) whereas only small amounts of 4-hydroxy-clobazam (M7) and 4-hydroxy-desmethyl-clobazam (M5) are detected after oral administration.

Up to the 97% of the dose is eliminated in the urine with only about 2% as unchanged drug. The main metabolite in the urine is M7, which is rapidly transformed into M9 (Volz et al., 1979).

Bibliography

Arendt RM, Greenblatt DJ, Liebish DC, Luu MD and Paul SM: Determinants of benzodiazepine brain uptake: lipophilicity versus binding affinity. *Psychopharmacology* 93:72-76, 1987

Divoll M, Greenblatt DJ, Ciraulo DA, Puri SK, Ho I and Shader RI: Clobazam kinetics: intrasubject variability and effect of food absorption. *Journal of Clinical Pharmacology* 22:69-73, 1982

Greenblatt DJ, Divoll M, Puri SK, Ho I, Zinny MA and Shader RI: Clobazam kinetics in the elderly. *British Journal of Clinical Pharmacology* 12:631-636, 1981

Rupp W, Badian M, Christ O et al.: Pharmacokinetics of single and multiple doses of clobazam in humans. *British Journal of Clinical Pharmacology* 7(suppl 1): 51S-57S, 1979

Vallner JJ, Needham TE, Jun HW, et al.: Plasma levels of clobazam after three oral dosage forme in healthy subjects. *Journal of Clinical Pharmacology* 18:319-324, 1978

Volz M, Christ O, Kellner H-M, et al.: Kinetics and metabolism of clobazam in animals and man. *British Journal of Clinical Pharmacology* 7(suppl 1):41S-50S, 1979

Clonazepam

CLONAZEPAM

After oral administration, its absorption is slow and nearly complete. Peak plasma concentrations are seen in 3-12 hours in fasting subjects and 82-98% of oral dose is detected in plasma (Boxenbaum et al., 1978).

Assuming complete oral bioavailability or after intravenous administration, the distribution volume of clonazepam has been calculated as approximately 1.59 l/kg (Eschenhof, 1973). It is 83-87% bound to serum albumin.

Clonazepam is extensively metabolized in the liver. The principal metabolite is the 7-amino-clonazepam produced by a reduction of the 7-nitro group. This is further converted by an acetylation process to 7-acetamido-clonazepam. Hydroxylation of both clonazepam and 7-amino-clonazepam to yield 3-OH and 7-amino-3-hydroxy-clonazepam respectively, represents a minor catabolic pathway (Eschenhof, 1973).

Clonazepam has a mean elimination half-life ranging between 25 and 48 hours. Metabolites are excreted in the urine and about 10-26% of the amount absorbed is found in the faeces. The rate of metabolism and excretion of clonazepam and its metabolites is significantly reduced by advancing age (Boxenbaum et al., 1978).

Bibliography

Boxenbaum HG, Posmanter HN, Macasieb T, Geitner KA, Weinfeld RE, Moore JD, Darragh A, O'Kelly DA, Weissman L and Kaplan SA: Pharmacokinetics of flunitrazepam following single and multiple dose oral administration to healthy subjects. *Journal of Pharmacology and Biopharmac* 6:283-293, 1978

Eschenhof E: Investigation of the fate of the anticonvulsivant clonazepam in rat, dog and man. *Arzneim Forsch* 23:390-400, 1973

Clorazepate

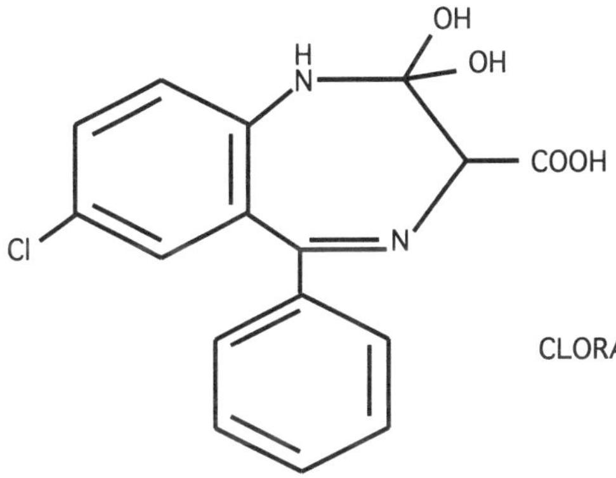

OH
H
N
OH
COOH
Cl
N
CLORAZEPATE

Clorazepate is a pro-drug for desmethyldiazepam. In fact, in the acid environment of the stomach it is converted by hydroxylation and a rapid decarbossilation to desmethyldiazepam, which is then almost completely absorbed (Greenblatt, 1978).

Desmethyldiazepam reaches peak plasma concentration in 1.9 hours following oral administration. However, its absorption is delayed in the presence of clorazepate. The distribution volume has been calculated to be about 1.11 ± 0.18 l/Kg (Aymard, 1978).

N-desmethyldiazepam is hydroxylated to form oxazepam which, in turn, is conjugated with glucuronic acid to be eliminated in the urine (Bertler, 1978).

Bibliography

Aymard N: Analyse pharmacocinetique d'une benzodiazepine, le clorazepate dipotassique. *Psychol Med* 10:145-154, 1978

Bertler A: Les aspects pharmacocinetiques des traitements par les benzodiazepines. *Psychol Med* 10:131141, 1978

Greenblatt DJ: Determination of desmethyldiazepam in plasma by electron-capture GLC: Application to pharmacokinetic studies of clorazepate. *Journal of Pharmaceutical Sciences* 67:427-429, 1978

Clotiazepam

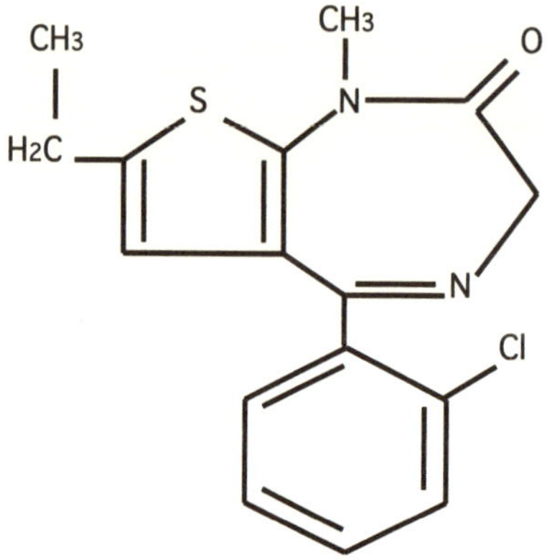

CLOTIAZEPAM

Clotiazepam is rapidly absorbed. Peak plasma levels are detected 0.5-1.5 hours after oral ingestion. The oral bioavailability of clotiazepam averages 25% because of its first pass through the liver. Its apparent distribution volume is 3.5 l/Kg, irrespective of a multiple dose schedule.

The mean half-life of clotiazepam elimination in humans is 3.7 hours, with considerable interindividual variations ranging from 2 to 5.6 hours. Following repeated oral administration (16 doses), the mean elimination half life is longer (4.9 hours) with a range of 2.9-6.7 hours (Bourin, 1989).

Clotiazepam is extensively protein bound with a free fraction in plasma of approximately 1%. Using the Scatchard equation to analyse binding data, it has been possible to identify two different binding sites with different affinities (Arendt et al., 1982).

Clotiazepam metabolism involves a hydroxylation and dealkylation process. The pharmacokinetics of these derivatives parallel those of the parent molecule.

Clotiazepam is not detectable in the urine, where the mono alcohol of the desmethyl-derivative is present, mainly in form of glucuron-conjugate.

Bibliography

Arendt R, Ochs HR and Greenblatt DJ: Electron capture GLC analysis of the thienodiazepine clotiazepam. *Arzneim Forsch* (Drug Res) 32:453-455, 1982

Bourin M: Pharmacocinetique des benzodiazepines In: *Les benzodiazepines: de la pharmacocinetique a la dependance.* Bourin M (ed.) Ellipses, Paris, pp. 31-88, 1989

Diazepam

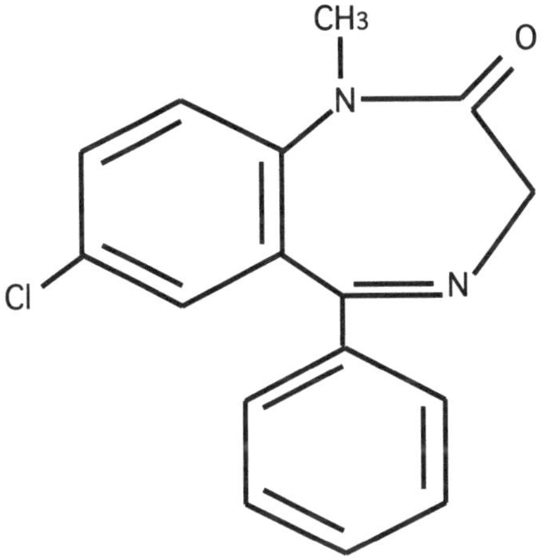

CH3 O N Cl N

DIAZEPAM

Following oral administration, diazepam is completely and rapidly absorbed, yielding peak plasma concentrations in 15-90 minutes in adults and in 15-30 minutes in children. A second peak is observed 6-12 hours later, probably due to enterohepatic recirculation (Mandelli et al., 1978).

After intramuscular injection, absorption is slow and erratic—but complete, with serum levels peaking after 10-12 hours (Gamble et al., 1975). When diazepam is rectally administered, its absorption is slow and inferior to that obtained by the oral route. Peak plasma levels are detected after 2-4 hours and the plasma concentrations are only 50% of those yielded by the same dose orally administered. 1 mg of diazepam/Kg given rectally to children results in a concentration of 270-320 μg/l after 5 minutes, while peak levels ranging between 600-1300 μg/l, are reached into 10-60 minutes. This suggests that in children the rectal route results in a rapid but not precisely predictable absorption (Meberg et al., 1978).

Following intravenous injection, effective plasma levels are reached in 15-30 seconds (Baird and Hailey, 1972). Due to the ripartition process, these concentrations decline after 30-60 minutes to reach those yielded after the equivalent oral dose (Klotz et al.,1976).

Diazepam is largely and quickly distributed through the body — which is to be expected of a highly lipophilic drug. The apparent distribution volume is approximately 1.1 l/Kg, suggesting extensive plasma albumin binding (98-99%) concentrations of diazepam in the CSF parallel those of the unbound drug in the plasma (Colburn and Gibaldi, 1978).

It passes into the breast milk of feeding mothers, and easily crosses the placenta. The ratio fetal/maternal plasma concentrations fluctuate with the time of the pregnancy and with the duration of the treatment. Following a single oral dose, it ranges from 1.2 in the first months to 1.8 at the end of the pregnancy. But it may vary from 0.4 at beginning to 0.8 in the last weeks of the pregnancy, when repeated doses are administered (Moore and McBride, 1978). However, since in the fetus and in the new born, diazepam is less largely bound to plasma proteins and the active free fraction is close to the 18%, this can easily induce toxic effects.

Diazepam is metabolized in the liver, where it produces three active metabolites:

- Desmethyldiazepam (or nordiazepam) which exhibits similar pharmacological properties to diazepam with a longer half-life. The mean plasma half-life is 30 hours with a range of 20-100 hours for diazepam, whereas for desmethyldiazepam mean plasma half-life ranges between 30-200 hours. During the beta phase, N-desmethyldiazepam serum concentrations exceed those of diazepam, either after single or multiple dose treatment.
- Hydroxylation of desmethyldiazepam produces oxazepam with a mean half-life of 9 hours (ranging from 5 to 15 hours). Oxazepam is excreted from the body after its conjugation with glucuronic acid.
- Temazepam is yielded by direct hydroxylation of diazepam. It displays a mean plasma half life of 12 hours (ranging from 10 to 20 hours). Temazepam may be directly conjugated with glucuronic acid before excretion or converted to oxazepam by dealkilation. Oxazepam and temazepam do not appear to significantly contribute to the pharmacodinamic effect because they possess shorter half-lives than the parent molecule.

Diazepam metabolism takes place extensively in the liver, while the metabolites are eliminated mainly through the kidneys. Metabolism and excretion of diazepam and its derivatives are age-dependent (Klotz et al., 1975). Plasma half-life can be over one week in patients aged 65. Elimination and biotransformation are impaired in the presence of severe liver and kidney diseases. However, a slower catabolism does not necessarily represent a serious problem because diazepam has a wide therapeutic index and N-desmethyl diazepam displays a longer half-life than the parent molecule (Mandelli et al., 1978).

Bibliography

Baird ES and Hailey DM: Delayed recovery from a sedative: correlation of the plasma levels of diazepam with clinical effects after oral and intravenous administration. *British Journal of Anaesthesiology* 44:803-808, 1972

Colburn WA and Gibaldi M: Plasma protein binding of diazepam after a single dose of sodium oleate. *Journal of Pharmaceutical Sciences* 67:891-892, 1978

Gamble JAS, Daundee JW and Assar RAE: Plasma diazepam levels after single dose oral and intramuscular administration. *Anesthesia* 30:164-169, 1975

Klotz U, Antonin KH and Bieck PR: Comparison of the pharmacokinetics of diazepam after single and subchronic doses. *European Journal of Clinical Pharmacology* 10:121-126, 1976

Klotz U, Avant GR, Hoyumpa A, Schenkers and Wilkinson GR: The effects of age and liver disease on the disposition and elimination of diazepam in adult man. *Journal of Clinical Investigation* 55:347-359, 1975

Mandelli M, Tognoni G and Garattini S: Clinical pharmacokinetics of diazepam. *Clinical Pharmacokinetics* 3:72-91, 1978

Meberg A, Langslet A, Bredesen JE and Lunde PKM: Plasma concentration of diazepam and Ndesmethyldiazepam in children after a single rectal or intramuscular dose of diazepam. *European Journal of Clinical Pharmacology* 14:273-276, 1978

Moore RG and Mc Bride WG: The disposition kinetics of diazepam in pregnant women at parturition. *European Journal of Pharmacology* 13:275-284, 1978

Flunitrazepam

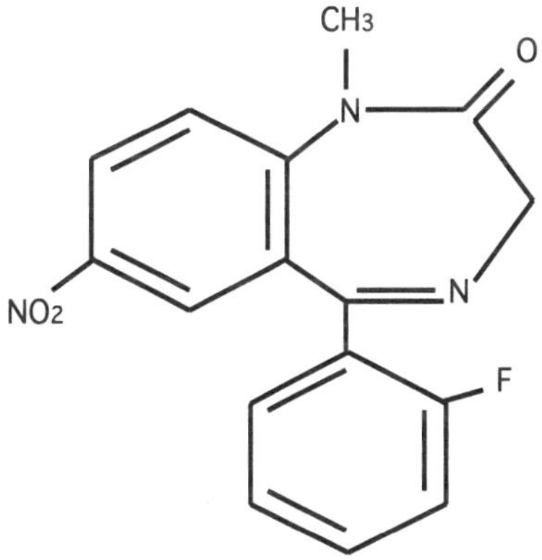

CH_3 O N N NO_2 F

FLUNITRAZEPAM

Flunitrazepam belongs to the 7-nitro-BDZs, and chemically it is close to nitrazepam and clonazepan. Absorption is rapid with Cmax obtained within 1-1.5 hours after oral doses. The estimated constant of absorption (Ka) is 1.9 ± 0.5 h^{-1}. The calculated bioavailability is about 89.5 ± 10.5%. Drug distribution is complete.

Following an intravenous injection, the profile of the curve showing drug plasma levels over time goes through three phases: a) rapid distribution; b) slow distribution; and c) the elimination phase. The distribution volume ranges from 2.2 to 4.1 l/Kg. The equation expression of this curve is three-esponential, and is related to flunitrazepam distribution in three compartments. After administration into the first compartment, flunitrazepam rapidly diffuses into the second compartment where it reaches a state of equilibrium in approximately 2 hours. The drug moves more slowly into the third compartment, larger than the other two, and reaches peak levels almost 17 hours after administration. The equilibrium state among the three compartments is reached in about twenty hours. By then, most of the flunitrazepam is in compartment three. This may account for the long half-life: the mean distribution half life is 3 ± 0.8 hours while the mean elimination half life is 21.5 ± 1.7 hours (Amrein et al., 1976; Singlas, 1979).

Some 80% of flunitrazepam in the blood is carried bound to plasma proteins.

It is widely metabolized in the liver and only 2% of the unchanged drug is recovered in the urine. The main metabolites generated are:

a) the 7-amino derivative yielded through a reduction of the 7-nitro group
b) 1-desmethyl-flunitrazepam obtained through a dealkyl reaction at position 1.
c) the derivative formed by an hydroxylation at position 3.

The presence of an hydroxy group allows a rapid glucurono conjugation. These metabolites undergo biotransformation to yield at least derivatives identified in the urine.

The time course of plasma concentration of both flunitrazepam and its metabolites shows that flunitrazepam, as an unchanged molecule, is the dominant drug during the first 8 hours following administration. The mean half-lives of 1-desmethyl-flunitrazepam and 7-amino derivative are 31 ± 8 and 23 ± 4 hours respectively (Wendt, 1976).

Clinical studies have demonstrated that the hypnotic effect of flunitrazepam is associated with plasma concentrations ranging between 6 and 8 ng/ml. After a single oral dose, these plasma levels are obtained in 30 minutes and last for at least 8 hours. Thus, there is a clear relationship between the time course of flunitrazepam plasma levels and its clinical effects.

Flunitrazepam and its derivatives are excreted essentially through the renal route (>90%) (Amrein et al., 1976). The flunitrazepam plasma elimination has a total clearance equal to 130 ± 11 ml/min. This clearance is hepatic, 98% of flunitrazepam metabolism takes place in the liver. On the basis of these data, it is advisable to reduce the daily dose of flunitrazepam where the liver function is seriously impaired.

During chronic treatment at 2 mg/day of flunitrazepam, peak plasma concentrations at steady-state are 10-12 ng/ml 2 hours after the treatment is started, a little higher than those yielded after a single dose. This may be explained by the distribution volume of the drug, and it may suggest that the hypnotic effect of flunitrazepam is not reduced by prolonged treatment.

Bibliography

Amrcin R, Cano JP and Hugin W: Pharmacokinetishe und pharmakodynamishebefunde nach einnaliger intravenoser, intramusculer und oraler applikation von Rohypnol. In: *Bisherige erfahrungen mit Rohypnol (flunitrazepam) in des anasthesiologie und intensivtherapie, Roche Edit.* Basel (Switzerland), pp. 39-56, 1976

Singlas E: Pharmacocinetique du flunitrazepam. *Nouvelle Presse Medicale* 8(suppl):2519-2523, 1979

Wendt G: Schicksel des hypnotikum flunitrazepam ins menschlichen organismum. In: *Bisherige erfahrungen mit Rohypnol (flunitrazepam) in des anasthesiologie und intensiv therapie, Roche Edit.* Basel (Switzerland), pp. 27-38, 1976

Flurazepam

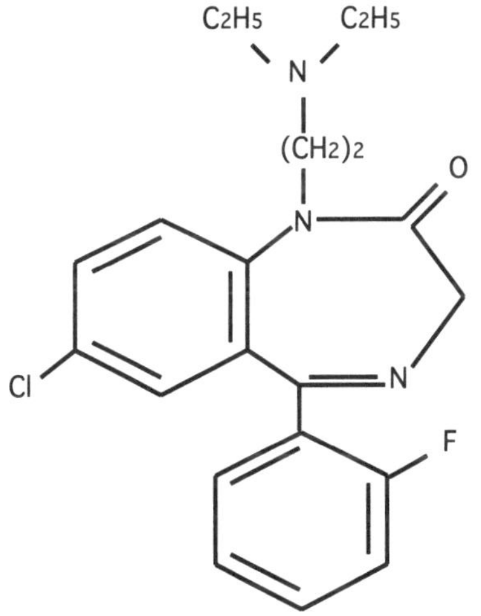

FLURAZEPAM

Flurazepam is absorbed rapidly and completely. Its bioavailability is 100%. Only negligible amounts of flurazepam can be measured in the plasma, since it is quickly converted to N-desalkyl flurazepam and N_1 (2-hydroxyethyl) flurazepam. These derivatives have elimination half-lives of 48-101 hours and 9-21 hours respectively. The parent drug itself possesses a half-life of only 2-3 hours. Peak serum levels are 11-22 μg/l three hours after a single oral dose, whereas the N-desalkyl derivative reaches 10 μg/l after 24 hours prolonged treatment, resulting in an accumulation of the active metabolites, mainly the N-desalkyl metabolite (Kaplan et al., 1973).

Flurazepam is largely bound to plasma protein, 98%. Its metabolites, N-desalkyl flurazepam and N_1 (2-hydroxyethyl) flurazepam are bound for 98% and 90% respectively. Flurazepam metabolism takes place in the liver and only a small fraction occurs in the gut. 58% of the dose is excreted in the urine with about 42% of the dose as N_1 (2-hydroxyethyl) derivative conjugated with glucuronic or sulphoric acid. Nine percent is eliminated with faeces (Breimer, 1977).

On the basis of its pharmacokinetics, flurazepam appears to be a long acting sleep inducer, with unequivocal residual effects present during next day (and sometimes appreciable the next evening). This is due to the marked accumulation of active metabolites with long half-life.

Although there is no evidence of a direct correlation between flurazepam serum levels and its clinical effect, liver and renal diseases seem to prolong action and potentiate the effect. Minor dosage and caution are therefore needed in using flurazepam to treat patients with sleep disorders, as well as the elderly (Greenblatt et al., 1975).

Bibliography

Breimer DD: Clinical pharmacokinetics of hypnotics. *Clinical Pharmacokinetics* 2:93-109, 1977

Greenblatt DJ, Shader RI and Koch-Weser J: Flurazepam hydrochloride. *Clinical Pharmacology and Therapeutics* 17:1-14, 1975

Kaplan SA, de Silva JAF, Jack ML, et al.: Blood level profile in man following chronic oral administration of flurazepam hydrochloride. *Journal of Pharmaceutical Sciences* 62:1932-1935, 1973

Ketazolam

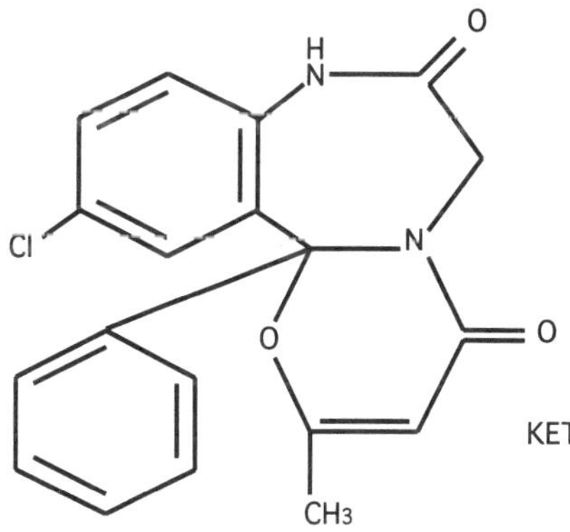

KETAZOLAM

Ketazolam is completely absorbed following an oral dose: its bioavailability is 100%. Peak plasma concentrations (4 μg/l) are yielded within 2 hours (Norman and Burrows, 1984; Eberts et al., 1977). As with other BDZ compounds, it is extensively bound to serum albumin.

Ketazolam is largely metabolized in the liver, and is rapidly converted into N-desmethyl-ketazolam and N-desmethyl-diazepam, each with plasma half-lives of 50 hours. Significant levels of these active metabolites are detectable in the plasma in the presence of negligible amounts of the unchanged parent molecule — whose mean half-life is very short, approximately 1.5 hours.

Oxazepam is the final product of the main metabolic pathway. 80% of a single oral dose of 30 mg of ketazolam is recovered in the urine as oxazepam or its glucuronic-conjugate, 20% is excreted with faeces.

According to the pharmacokinetic parameters, it is likely that the biological activity displayed by ketazolam when administered once a day is actually exercised by its desmethyl derivatives. Moreover, diazepam is measurable in the plasma after a single oral 30 mg dose of ketazolam. Diazepam is also converted to N-desmethyldiazepam, which may explain why the clinical profile of ketazolam resembles that of diazepam (Kabra et al., 1978).

Bibliography

Eberts FS, Philopoulos Y, Reineke LM, Vliek RW and Metxler CN: Disposition of ketazolam, a new anxiolytic agent. *Pharmacologist* 19:165, 1977

Kabra PM, Stevens GL and Marton LJ: High pressure liquid chromatography analysis of diazepam, oxazepam and N-desmethyldiazepam in human blood. *Journal of Chromatography* 150:355-360, 1978

Norman TR and Burrows GD: Plasma concentrations of benzodiazepines—a review of clinical findings and implications. *Progress in Neuropharmacology and Biological Psychiatry* 8:115-126, 1984

Loprazolam

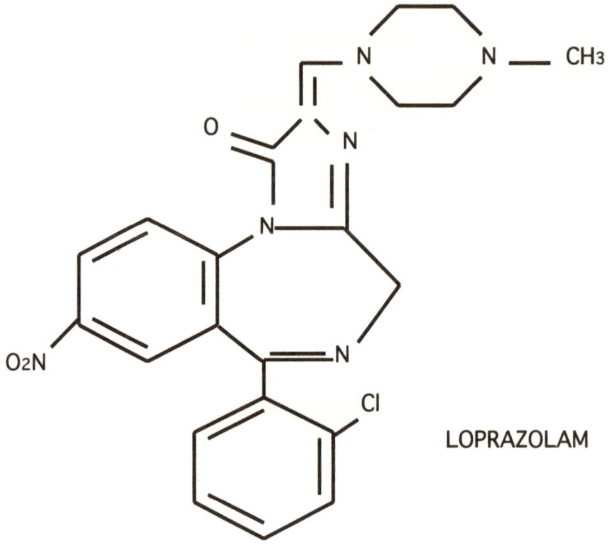

LOPRAZOLAM

Loprazolam is a 1,4 imidazolebenzodiazepine, with a basic heterocycle ring at the 1,2 position of the diazepine ring. It also possesses: a) a nitro group at position 8 on the diazepine nucleus, b) a carboxy group at position 1 on the fused imidazole nucleus and c) a piperazine ring at position 2 of the imidazole ring system.

The presence of the imidazole ring means it is possible to make preparations of aqueous injectable solutions that are stable and well tolerated. Loprazolam is well absorbed after oral administration. Peak plasma concentration occurs 0.5-3 hours after a morning dose in fasting subjects and 2-4.5 hours after night time doses in non-fasting subjects (Stevens et al., 1983; McInnes et al., 1985). Peak levels on day 8 are not statistically different from those detected on day 1. Tmax is similar on the first day and after 8 days.

Age, gender and body weight do not seem to affect the absorption characteristics of loprazolam.

Its estimated system bioavailability is 70% of an oral dose. The volume of distribution is large, ranging from 2.83 to 31.5 l/kg, with great interindividual variations. The plasma protein binding of loprazolam is approximately 80% (Illing et al., 1983).

In one third of lactating women who take a single dose of loprazolam, traces of drug are found in the breast-milk 2 and 12 hours later (0.9 and 2.9 μg/l respectively). The transfer of loprazolam is still unexplored in vivo placental. However, in vitro investigations using artificial perfusion of human placenta indicate that loprazolam is easily able to cross the placental barrier without being fixed by the tissue, whereas both diazepam and clorazepate are reported to accumulate in the placenta.

Loprazolam does not metabolize rapidly. The major elimination pathway involves the N-oxidation of the piperazine ring. Minor metabolites are the hydroxy loprazolam (accounting for 3%), the acetamido-loprazolam (less than 4%) and loprazolam-conjugate derivatives (almost 25%) (Illing et al., 1983).

The elimination half-life of loprazolam ranges from 4 to 7 hours, making it an intermediate-acting BDZ, and this is not affected by the time of day of administration, or by the sex of the patient. However, there is a slight delay after multiple doses, even if this has no statistical significance. A trend toward a more prolonged half-life is observed in the elderly. This may arise from differences in distribution volume or may reflect changes in the rates of metabolic elimination occurring with age (Swift, 1983; Stevens et al., 1985).

The actual impact of kidney and liver illness on the pharmacokinetics of loprazolam remains to be investigated. Although loprazolam interaction with commonly used drugs has not been extensively explored, it is reasonable to expect that substances able to affect the microsomial liver enzyme system could modify loprazolam pharmacokinetics.

Bibliography

Illing HPA, Ings RMJ, Johnson KI and Fromson JM: Disposition of ^{14}C-loprazolam in animals and man. *Xenobotica* 13:439-449, 1983

McInnes GT, Bunting EA, Ings RMJ, Robinson J and Ankier SI: Pharmacokinetics and pharmacodynamics following single and repeated nightly administrations of loprazolam, a new benzodiazepine hypnotic. *British Journal of Clinical Pharmacology* 19:649-656, 1985

Stevens LA, Bevan CD, Salmon J, Krieger J, Perianu M, et al.: Single and repeated dose kinetics of the hypnotic agent loprazolam in healthy volunteers. *European Journal of Clinical Pharmacology* 25:651-655, 1983

Stevens LA, Pidgen, AW, Bevan CD, Ings RMJ, Lawrence JR, et al.: Correlation of the clinical pharmacodynamics of loprazolam with serum concentration. *Xenobiotica* 15:623-631, 1985

Swift CG: Pharmacokinetics and pharmacodynamics of loprazolam in the young and elderly. Loprazolam Clinical Workshop, Florence Italy, Medicine Publishing Foundation, Oxford pp.10, 1983

Lorazepam

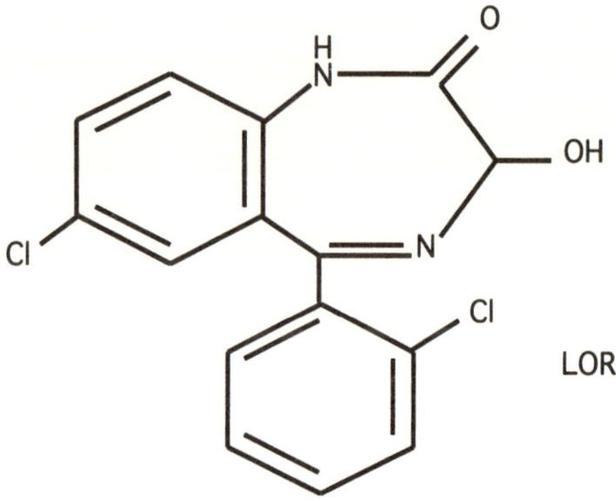

LORAZEPAM

Lorazapam is structurally very close to oxazepam. It is almost completely absorbed through the gastrointestinal tract. Its oral bioavailability averages 90%. Lorazepam peak plasma concentrations are obtained 2 hours after oral ingestion.

After the administration per os, a "lag period", ranging from 15 to 30 minutes, is observed, in which drug plasma levels are below the sensitivity limit of analytical methods. A slow crossing through the gastric and proximal tract of duodenal mucuses may account for this phenomenon (Ka = 2.75 h^{-1}). The estimated volume of distribution ranges between 1.14-1.33 l/kg. The total plasma clearance appears to be 1.05-1.10 ml/min/kg. The elimination half-life is 14.1 ± 3.7 hours, irrespective of dose and administration route (Greenblatt et al., 1979).

Lorazepam in the blood is bound to plasma proteins in the proportion of 65-75% (Greenblatt, 1981). It possesses a longer duration of action than its half-life would suggest. The extent of its binding affinity to the brain receptor sites correlates with its duration of action. However, in spite of its lack of active metabolites, there is no direct correlation between drug serum concentration and its clinical effect (Spirt et al., 1981).

Lorazepam is completely metabolized in the liver: only 0.5% of the unchanged drug is recovered in the urine. The hepatic biotransformation involves conjugation at position 3 with glucuronic acid. This reaction produces a water soluble, inactive derivative which is excreted in the urine. 75% of the dose is recovered in the urine in the form of glucuronic-conjugate. Other minor metabolites (including hydroxy-lorazepam, quinoline and quinolinine derivatives) have some importance in other animal species, but not in humans.

In addition, unlike the situation with many other BDZs, the metabolites are not involved in determining any pharmacological effect. The accumulation of both lorazepam and its derivatives during prolonged treatment is negligible. Elimination proccss is terminated one week after the stop of lorazepam assumption (Ameer and Greenblatt, 1981).

Animal investigations show that five days after the administration of [^{14}C]-labelled lorazepam, more than 95.6% of radioactivity is recovered in the urine. 75% of this activity is related to lorazepam glucuronide-conjugate and 19.4% to the minor metabolites. Small amounts are only detectable in the faeces in the first 3 days. The renal elimination of the labelled drug is almost complete after 4 days. It cannot be ruled out that an enterohepatic cycle may exist for some minor metabolites (Greenblatt et al., 1976).

In the light of its pharmacokinetics, the use of lorazepam is advisable in the elderly, as well as in conditions of liver impairment. The conjugation process is unaffected by age and liver diseases. Renal insufficiency may slow the elimination of its glucuronide-conjugate, but this has no pharmacological consequences, since this derivative lacks any activity.

Bibliography

Ameer B and Greenblatt DJ: Lorazepam, a review of its clinical pharmacological properties and therapeutic uses. *Drugs* 21:161-200, 1981

Greenblatt DJ: Clinical pharmacokinetics of oxazepam and lorazepam. *Clinical Pharmacokinetics* 6:89-105, 1981

Greenblatt DJ, Schillings RT, Kyriakopoulos AA et al.: Clinical pharmacokinetics of lorazepam. I Absorption and disposition of oral ^{14}C-lorazepam. *Clinical Pharmacology and Therapeutics* 20:329-341, 1976

Greenblatt DJ, Shader RI, Franke K, et al.: Pharmacokinetics and bioavailability of intravenous, intramuscular and oral lorazepam in humans. *Journal of Pharmaceutical Sciences* 68:57-63, 1979

Spirt NM, Bautz G, Zanko M, Horst WD and O'Brien RA: Comparative receptor binding effects in brain after i.v. lorazepam and diazepam administration. *Society of Neuroscience Abstract* 7:865, 1981

Midazolam

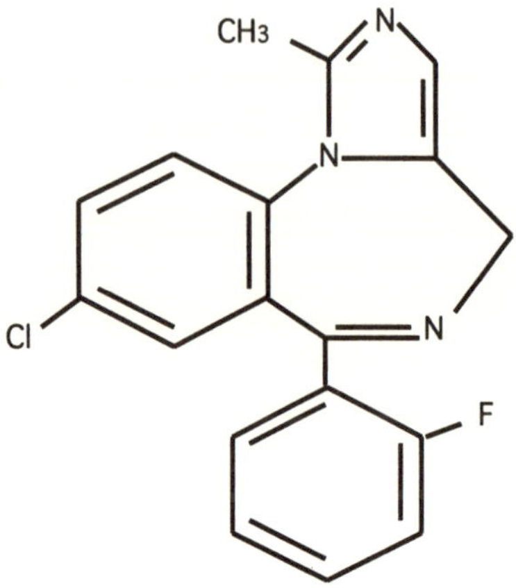

MIDAZOLAM

Midazolam is an imidazolo-benzodiazepine. The fused imidazolo ring protects it against hydrolysis, thus delaying degradation and loss of potency.

At physiological pH, midazolam becomes very lipophilic which contributes to a rapid absorption in the gastrointestinal tract. Peak plasma concentrations occur in 20-60 minutes following an oral dose. By using a compartmental analysis approach, the estimated absorption half-life is 14 minutes. For midazolam, a non linear correlation between dosage and plasma concentrations is described as 7.5 mg, 15 mg and 39 mg yield 34 μg/l, 60 μg/l and 220 μg/l respectively.

As with all BDZs, the rate and the extent of absorption decreases when the drug is co-administered with or ingested one hour after meals. Systemic bioavailability after oral administration ranges between 31 and 72%, due to the high liver extraction. Midazolam is almost completely absorbed following intramuscular injection, appearing in the systemic circulation within 5 minutes, while peak plasma levels are obtained within 20-30 minutes. After intramuscular injection, the systemic bioavailability ranges between 82 and 91% of the absolute bioavailability.

Following intravenous injection, it is rapidly and widely distributed, with a steady-state distribution volume ranging between 0.8-1.7 l/Kg. Considerable intersubject variations have been reported.

Smoking and gender do not affect the distribution volume, but evidence of the influence of age is conflicting. In healthy subjects, midazolam displays a short distribution phase half-life of between 5 and 30 minutes (Heizmann et al., 1983).

The kinetics are well described by a two compartment model within an elimination half-life of 2-3 hours. Age is believed to prolong this parameter.

Between 94-98% of midazolam is bound to plasma proteins (Dundee et al., 1984). Thus, small changes in plasma protein concentrations may induce relatively large variations in the levels of available unbound molecule, resulting in important effects on pharmacological activity. The free fraction is significantly higher in patients with renal insufficiency, whereas age, body weight and gender do not alter the protein binding of midazolam (Vinik et al., 1983).

Maternal and fetal midazolam plasma concentrations have been evaluated in several studies on women undergoing elective caesarian surgery, and where a premedication dose of 0.5 mg/Kg was intramuscularly injected. Midazolam concentration ratios between maternal and umbilical blood have been reported to be 1.27 and 2.15 for venous and arterial fetal blood respectively (Kanto et al., 1984).

The biotransformation of midazolam takes place in the liver. It undergoes hydroxylation and subsequent glucuronidation. The major derivative is α-hydroxy midazolam, which is pharmacologically active but less so than the parent drug. The elimination half-life of this metabolite is approximately one hour, while midazolam elimination half life ranges between 1 and 2.5 hours. Alpha-hydroxy midazolam may participate in the pharmacological activity of the parent drug after oral administration (Gerecke, 1983). Small amounts of 4-hydroxy midazolam and 1,4-dihydroxy midazolam are also generated, and excreted in the urine as glucuronide derivatives (Crevoisier et al., 1983).

Midazolam is oxidized by a member of the P450 III_A subfamily and thus its plasma concentrations may be reduced if microenzymatic inducers, such as macrolide antibiotics and phenytoin are coadministered.

The metabolites of midazolam have been observed during a period of liver transplantation, suggesting that an extra hepatic site of drug metabolism exists (Park et al., 1989).

Bibliography

Crevoisier CH, Ziegler WH, Eckert M and Heizman O: Relationship between plasma concentration and effect of midazolam after oral and intravenous administration. *British Journal of Clinical Pharmacology* 16:51S-61S, 1983

Dundee JW, Halliday NJ and Loughran PG: Variation in response to midazolam. *British Journal of Clinical Pharmacology* 17:645P-646P, 1984

Gerecke M: Chemical structure and properties of midazolam compared with other benzodiazepines. *British Journal of Clinical Pharmacology* 16:11S-16S, 1983

Heizmann P, Eckert M and Ziegler G: Pharmacokinetics and bioavailability of midazolam in man. *British Journal of Clinical Pharmacology* 16:43S-49S, 1983

Kanto J, Aaltonen L, Erkkola R and Aarimaa L: Pharmacokinetic and sedative effect of midazolam in connection with Caesarean section performed under epidural analgesía. *Acta Anaesthesiologica Scandinavica* 28:116-118, 1984
Park GR, Manara A and Dawling S: Extra-hepatic metabolism of midazolam. *British Journal of Clinical Pharmacology* 27:634-637, 1989
Vinik HR, Reves JG, Greenblatt DJ and Abernethy DR: Pharmacokinetics of midazolam in chronic renal failure patients. *Anesthesiology* 59:390-394, 1983

Nitrazepam

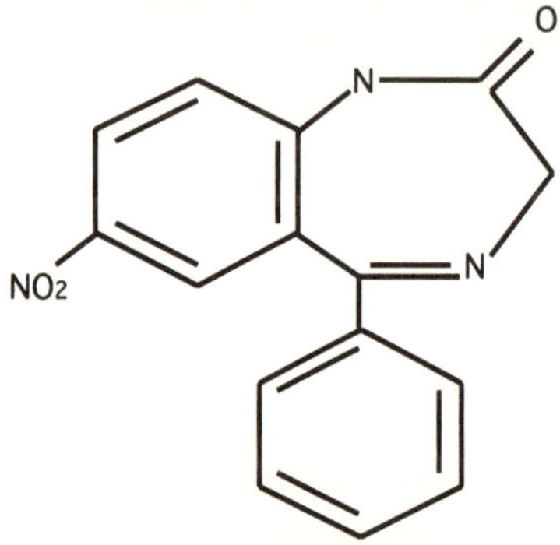

O
N
N
NO_2
NITRAZEPAM

Nitrazepam is readily absorbed from the gastrointestinal tract with a rapid penetration in the brain. Peak serum concentrations are obtained two hours after oral administration. The calculated absorption constant is $2.057\ h^{-1} < Ka < 2.219\ h^{-1}$. Mean systemic bioavailability is about 78% of the oral dose, with large intersubject variations ranging from 53% to 94% (Rieder and Wendt, 1973). The distribution phase is short, the decline in plasma levels being biphasic. The distribution volume, calculated after an intramuscular injection of 10 mg of drug, averages 1.95 l/Kg ranging from 1.45 to 2.80 l/Kg (Breimer et al., 1977). The mean nitrazepam half-life is 24 hours in young volunteers and 40 hours in the elderly, both under prolonged medication (5 mg/daily for two months). 87% of nitrazepam, circulating in the blood, is protein bound.

Entry into and egress from CSF are slow. But nitrazepam penetrates placenta quite rapidly, and fetal concentrations are similar to those found in maternal blood. During late pregnancy, placenta is easily permeable to nitrazepam in both directions. Equilibrium is reached 6 hours after oral administration. Traces of nitrazepam are detected in the breast-milk of feeding mothers: 5 mg/per os a day yields concentrations of 5-10 μg/100 ml of total drug (parent molecule and metabolites) in the breast-milk.

Nitrazepam is widely metabolized in the liver with only 4% of the dose excreted unchanged (Iisalo et al., 1977). The degradation process involves eduction of the nitro group to the corresponding amine with production of 7-amino-nitrazepam. This undergoes acetylation to yield the major metabolite, 7-acetoamido-nitrazepam. Hydroxylation at position 3 leads to the formation of 3-hydroxy-nitrazepam. Cleavage of the BDZ ring results in the generation of 2-amino-5-nitrobenzophenone and 2-amino-3-hydroxy-5-nitrophenone. Only nitrazepam is biologically active. Steady-state concentration is reached after 4 days.

Nitrazepam-derivatives are eliminated in the urine and almost 20% of an oral dose is found in the faeces (Beyer, 1971).

Bibliography

Beyer KH: La biotransformation des derives de la benzodiazepine Traduit de l'allemand: *Deutsche Apoteker Zeitung* 3:1503-1506, 1971

Breimer DD, Bracht H and de Boer AG: Plasma level profile of nitrazepam following oral administration. *British Journal of Clinical Pharmacology* 4:709, 1977

Iisalo E, Kangas L and Ruikka I: Pharmacokinetics of nitrazepam in young volunteers and aged patients. *British Journal of Clinical Pharmacology* 4:646P-647P, 1977

Rieder J and Wendt G: Pharmacokinetic and metabolism of the hypnotic nitrazepam. In: *The benzodiazepines*. Garattini S, Mussini E and Randall LO (eds.), Raven Press, New York, pp. 99-127, 1973

Oxazepam

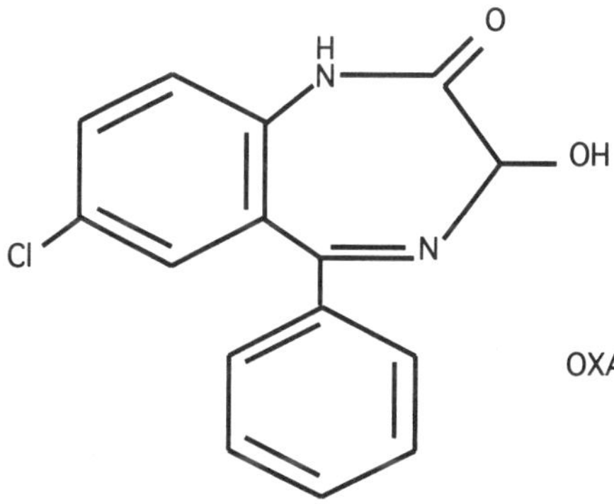

O
H
N
OH
Cl
N

OXAZEPAM

Oxazepam is completely absorbed after an oral dose. Peak plasma levels are reached 1-5 hours following its administration. There is a direct correlation between the doses and peak concentration, because they vary in the same direction according to a linear function. The bioavailability following oral administration averages 96%. Unlike other BDZs, oxazepam absorption is not significantly impaired when co-administered with meals. Since preparations for parental use are not available, the absolute bioavailability of oxazepam has not been determined. By using an oral form, the estimated distribution volume ranges from 0.4 to 2.3 l/Kg. The mean plasma half-life averages 9 hours, ranging from 3.7-21.2 hours. Between 87-96% of oxazepam in the blood is protein bound, with a free fraction ranging from 4 to 13% (Greenblatt, 1981).

Data on the oxazepam concentration in CSF and in brain tissue are not presently available. It is known that the drug is excreted in the breast-milk in small amounts, whereas it is found in the placental tissue in concentrations higher than those detected in the mother (Tomson et al., 1979).

Oxazepam is extensively metabolized in the liver. Very little amounts of the unchanged molecule are excreted. Excretion is primarily in the urine (67-80%) with 3-6% in the faeces after 3 days. Oxazepam biotransformation involves hepatic glucuronic acid conjugation, but a number of minor additional metabolites (including quinazolinone and hydroxy derivatives) have been identified. About 30% of the dose is metabolized during absorption in animals (Alvan et al., 1978).

Severe impairment of the liver function does not seem to significantly affect absorption, distribution, metabolism and the elimination rate of the drug and its derivatives (Shull et al., 1976). In patients with renal failure, the total clearance of oxazepam is similar to that calculated in normal subjects. However, the mean plasma elimination half-life is slower (ranging from 24 to 80 hours) and the free circulating fraction is higher (16%) (Odar-Cederloff et al., 1977). Age and gender do not influence oxazepam pharmacokinetics (Greenblatt et al., 1980).

Oxazepam does not possess a metabolite with biological activity — it is however, the active metabolite of many BDZs, including chlordiazepoxide, clorazepate, diazepam, ketazolam, medazepam, prazepam and temazepam. Steady-state concentrations are reached 2 days after multiple dose administration. There is a large range of intersubject variation in plasma steady-state levels following the oral administration of identical dose of oxazepam (Alvan et al., 1977).

Bibliograghy

Alvan G, Jonsson M, Sundwell A and Vessman J: First pass conjugation and enterohepatic recycling of oxazepam in dogs; intravenous tolerance of oxazepam in propylene glycol. *Acta Pharmacologica et Toxicologica* 40(suppl 1):16-27, 1978

Alvan G, Siwers B and Vessman J: Pharmacokinetics of oxazepam in healthy volunteers. *Acta Pharmacologica et Toxicologica* 40(suppl 1):40-51, 1977
Greenblatt DJ: Clinical pharmacokinetics of oxazepam and lorazepam. *Clinical Pharmacokinetics* 6:89-105, 1981
Greenblatt DJ, Divoll M, Harmatz JS and Shader RI: Oxazepam kinetics: effects of age and sex. *Journal of Pharmacology and Experimental Therapeutics* 215:86-91, 1980
Odar-Cederloff I, Vessman J, Alvan G and Sjoqvist F: Oxazepam disposition in uraemic patients. *Acta Pharmacologica et Toxicologica* 40(suppl 1):52-62, 1977
Shull HJ, Wilkinson GR, Johnson R and Shenker S: Normal disposition of oxazepam in acute viral hepatitis and cirrhosis. *Annals of Internal Medicine* 84:420-425, 1976
Tomson G, Lunell NO, Sundwall A and Rane A: Placent passage of oxazepam and its metabolism in mother and newborn. *Clinical Pharmacology and Therapeutics* 25:74-81, 1979

Prazepam

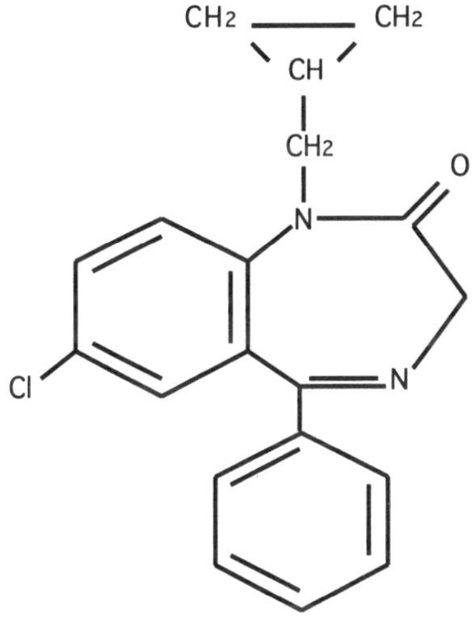

CH2 CH2
CH
CH2
O
N
Cl
N

PRAZEPAM

Prazepam is a pharmacologically inactive BDZ (Greenblatt and Shader, 1978a). Following oral administration, almost 90% of prazepam is absorbed, even if only small amounts of prazepam can be measured in the plasma. In fact, the drug undergoes almost complete pre-systemic biotransformation at hepatic level, generating its major derivative, desmethyldiazepam. Peak plasma concentrations of this active metabolite are reached within about 7 hours, with interindividual variations ranging from 3 to 41 hours. Desmethyldiazepam is extensively bound to plasma proteins (>97%) (Di Carlo et al., 1971).

Due to its high lipid solubility, it is readily and widely distributed through the body according to a model of two compartments. The estimated apparent distribution volume of desmethyl diazepam ranges from 0.5 to 2.5 l/Kg and this is increased by age, which leads to a slow half-life. Its mean plasma half-life averages 60 hours with significant individual variations ranging from 30 to 200 hours (Smith et al., 1979).

Prazepam is completely metabolized in the liver, so is undetectable in the urine (Di Carlo et al., 1969; Di Carlo and Viau, 1969). Biotransformation involves dealkylation forming desmethyl diazepam, which in turn, is hydroxylated to yield oxazepam (Di Carlo et al., 1971).

The elimination half-life of prazepam is expressed in terms of the elimination half-lives of its metabolites: an estimated 35 hours for the glucuronide conjugates and 120 hours for the non conjugate derivatives. The main metabolites are excreted in the urine as glucoronide conjugates (87.3% including both 3-hydroxyprazepam glucuronide and oxazepam glucoronide) (Allen et al., 1979).

According to prazepam pharmacokinetics, extensive accumulation of the active metabolites along prolonged multiple dose treatment can be expected. But the clinical effects of the drug do not seem to be similarly cumulative (Greenblatt and Shader, 1978b). The appearance of tolerance may account, at least partially, for this phenomenon.

In any case, the main question about prazepam use in therapy is if it is more reasonable to utilize prazepam per se or to directly administer its active metabolite.

Bibliography

Allen MD, Greenblatt DJ, Harmatz JS and Shader RI: Single dose kinetics of prazepam, a precursor of desmethyldiazepam. *Journal of Clinical Pharmacology* 19:445-450, 1979

Di Carlo FJ, Crew MC, Melgar MD and Haynes IJ: Prazepam metabolism by dogs. *Journal of Pharmaceutical Sciences* 58:960-962, 1969

Di Carlo FJ and Viau JP: Prazepam metabolites in dog urine. *Journal of Pharmaceutical Sciences* 59:322-325, 1969

Di Carlo FJ, Viau JP, Epps JE and Haynes LJ: Biotransformation of prazepam in man. *Annals of the New York Academy of Sciences* 178:487-492, 1971

Greenblatt DJ and Shader RI: Prazepam, a precursor of desmethyldiazepam. *Lancet* 2:270, 1978a

Greenblatt DJ and Shader RI: Pharmacokinetic understanding of anti-anxiety drug therapy. *Southern Medical Journal* 71S:3-9, 1978b

Smith HT, Evans LEJ, Eadie MJ and Typer JH: Pharmacokinetics of prazepam in man. *European Journal of Clinical Pharmacology* 16:141-147, 1979

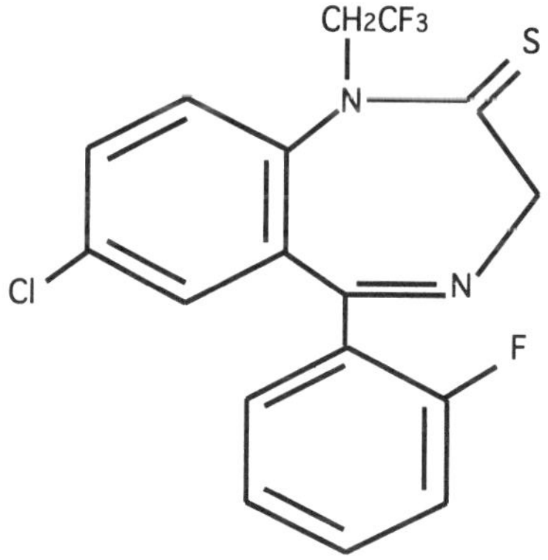

Quazepam

Quazepam is a trifluoroethyl-benzodiazepine which has been demonstrated to possess hypnotic properties. In addition to sedative-hypnotic effects, quazepam also displays anxiolytic, anticonvulsant and myorelaxant activities, characteristic of BDZ profiles.

Following oral administration, maximum quazepam plasma concentration is achieved in 2.4 hours (30 μg/l after a single dose of 15 mg) and seems to be subject to diurnal variations (Hilbert et al., 1984).

Quazepam is widely distributed in the body with an apparent volume of distribution of the central compartment of 5.0 l/Kg. In the blood, it is bound to plasma proteins in a proportion greater than 95%.

Quazepam is rapidly metabolized. The hepatic biotransformation involves substitution of the sulphur group with oxygen. This reaction produces the acid derivative 2-oxoquazepam (2-OQ) which is further metabolized either by hydroxylation to 3-hydroxy-2-oxoquazepam (3-HOQ) or by N-dealkylation to the pharmacologically inactive product N-desalkyl-2-oxoquazepam (DOQ) (Zampaglione et al., 1985). Although the brain concentration of this latter derivative is higher than the parent drugs, animal investigations show that hypnotic activity correlates better with quazepam and 2-OQ brain concentrations (Hilbert et al., 1986).

As the degradative pathway initially involves hepatic substitution, it is likely that drugs which induce (e.g. rifampin) or inhibit (e.g. anti-H_2, propranolol, oral contraceptives, disulfiram) the activity of liver microsomal oxidative enzymes affect quazepam metabolism. The half-life of this compound ranges between 27 and 40 hours after a single oral dose. Multiple dosing does not modify this kinetic parameter. DOQ, HOQ and HDOQ are further catabolized to inactive conjugates of glucuronic acid, before being excreted (Zampaglione et al., 1985).

The elimination half-lives of the two main metabolites are 40 hours for OQ and 70 hours for DOQ, respectively (Hilbert et al., 1984). The latter compound accumulates in the plasma (Chung et al., 1984). The clinical significance of this is still unclear, since the contribution of DOQ to the pharmacological activity of quazepam is not yet fully understood (Hilbert et al., 1986). Quazepam is slowly eliminated in the urine and faeces as derivatives, and only very negligible amounts of unchanged quazepam are detected (Zampaglione et al., 1985). About 0.2% passes into breast milk in 24 hours (Hilbert et al., 1984).

Quazepam administration, 15 mg by the oral route, at bedtime provides an hypnotic effect without significant side effects. 15 mg seems to be a dose which is both effective and well tolerated in the elderly, even though 7.5 mg appears more appropriate in the presence of age, or hepatic and renal dysfunction. Fatigue, drowsiness and daytime somnolence are the most frequent unwanted effects, which are predictable from its pharmacological profile. The incidence of the severity of these side-effects increases with doses. Unlike reference BDZs, quazepam induces ataxia very infrequently: its relative selectivity for the $omega_1$ receptor site may account for this (Corda et al., 1986).

Bibliography

Corda MG, Sanna E, Concas A, Giorgi O, Ongini E, et al.: Enhancement of gamma-aminobutyric acid binding by quazepam, a benzodiazepine derivative with preferential affinity for type I benzodiazepine receptors. *Journal of Neurochemistry* 42:370-374, 1986

Chung M, Hilbert JM, Gural RP, Radwanski E, Symchowicz S, et al.: Multi-dose quazepam kinetics. *Clinical Pharmacology and Therapeutics* 35:520-524, 1984

Hilbert JM, Chung M, Maier G, Gural R, Symchowicz S, et al.: Effect of sleep on quazepam kinetics. *Clinical Pharmacology and Therapeutics* 36:99-104, 1984

Hilbert JM, Gural RP, Symchowicz S and Zampaglione N: Excretion of quazepam into human breast milk. *Journal of Clinical Pharmacology* 24:457-462, 1984

Hilbert JM, Iorio L, Moritzen V, Barnett A, Symchowicz S, et al.: Relationship of brain and plasma levels of quazepam, flurazepam, and their metabolites with pharmacological activity in mice. *Life Sciences* 39:164-168, 1986

Zampaglione N, Hilbert JM, Ning J, Chung M, Gural R, et al.: Disposition and metabolic fate of ^{14}C-quazepam in man. *Drug Metabolism and Disposition* 13:25-29, 1985

Temazepam

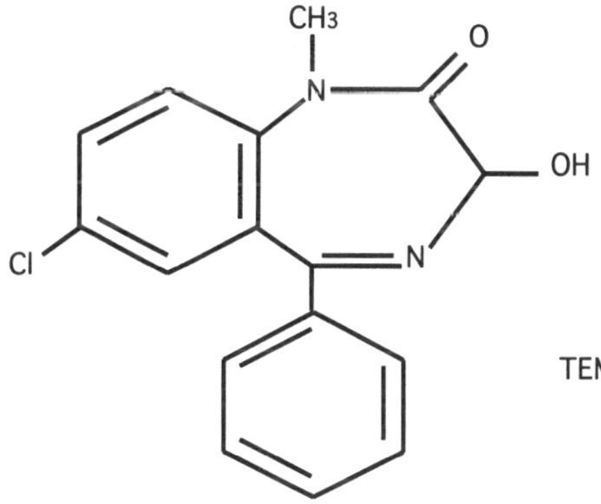

CH_3 O OH Cl N N

TEMAZEPAM

Temazepam is a member of the 1,4 benzodiazepine series. When administered orally, using gelatine capsules containing a solution of the drug in polyethylene glycol, it is rapidly and completely absorbed (Fucella, 1979). Peak plasma concentrations are obtained in less than 1 hour and at least 80% of this maximum concentration is reached within 20 minutes after the oral ingestion in fasting conditions (Patterson, 1986; Fucella et al., 1977).

Assuming complete oral bioavailability, the distribution volume of temazepam has been calculated as approximately 1.3-1.6 l/Kg (Fucella et al., 1972).

Temazepam circulates in the blood extensively bound to plasma proteins with a free fraction averaging 24% (Divoll et al., 1981). The alpha phase of diffusion has been estimated to range from 2 to 3 hours (Curry and Whelpton, 1979).

Temazepam is completely metabolized in the liver. It is converted to oxazepam through desmethylation, but this metabolic route accounts for only 5% of temazepam degradation. The main pathway involves a glucurono-conjugation of the parent drug. This derivative may undergo a desmethylation, which generates oxazepam-glucuronide conjugate. Elimination is essentially through the kidney (>80%), while faecal excretion accounts for 12% (Schwartz, 1979).

Reported elimination half-life values for temazepam range from 5.5 to 11.5 hours. Morning assumption of the drug seems to be associated to a 30% increase in elimination half-life (Bittencourt et al., 1979). Age appears to slightly slow the elimination half-life: the average is 15 hours in the elderly (Cook, 1980). The half-life in elderly women may be longer than in elderly men (Smith et al., 1983). There are no data currently available about the possibility of temazepam passing into breast-milk or crossing the placental barrier. However, judging by its structural similarity to other BDZs, it is likely to pass into both milk and the fetus.

Bibliography

Bittencourt P, Richens A, Toseland PA, Wicks JFC and Latham AN: Pharmacokinetics of the hypnotic benzodiazepine, temazepam. *British Journal of Clinical Pharmacology* 8:37S-38S, 1979

Cook P: Change in benzodiazepine drug activity with ageing In: *Current trends in therapeutics in the elderly*. Exton-Smith AN (ed.), Oxford Medical Education Services, pp. 23-32, 1980

Curry SH and Whelpton R: Pharmacokinetics of related benzodiazepines. *British Journal of Clinical Pharmacology* 8:15S-21S, 1979

Divoll M et al.: Effect of age and gender on the disposition of temazepam. *Journal of Pharmacological Science* 70:1104-1107, 1981

Fucella LM: Bioavailability of temazepam in soft gelatin capsules. *British Journal of Clinical Pharmacology* 8:31S-35S, 1979

Fucella LM, Bolcioni G, Tomassia V, Ferrario L and Tognoni G: Human pharmacokinetics and bioavailability of temazepam administered in soft gelatin capsules. *European Journal of Clinical Pharmacology* 12:383-386, 1977

Fucella LM, Tosolini G, Moro E and Tomassia V: Study of physiological availability of temazepam in man. *International Journal of Clinical Pharmacology* 6:303-309, 1972

Patterson SE: Determination of temazepam in plasma and urine by high performance liquid chromatography using disposable solid phase extraction columns. *Journal of Pharmaceutical and Biomedical Analysis* 4:271-274, 1986

Schwartz HJ: Pharmacokinetics and metabolism of temazepam in man and several animal species. *British Journal of Clinical Pharmacology* 8:23S-29S, 1979

Smith RB, Divoll M, Gillespie WR and Greenblatt DJ: Effect of subject age and gender on the pharmacokinetics of oral triazolam and temazepam. *Journal of Clinical Psychopharmacology* 3:172-176, 1983

Triazolam

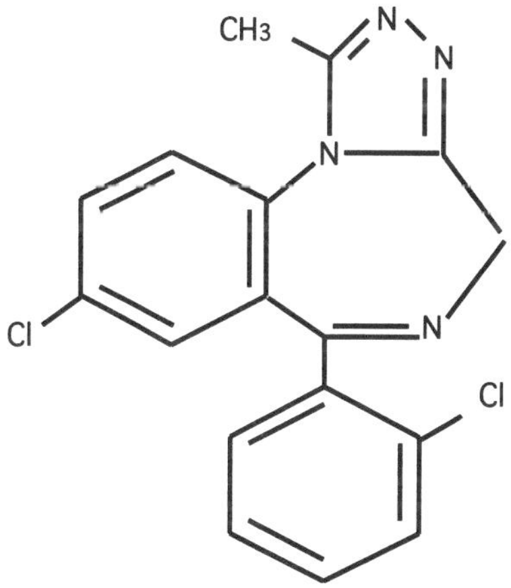

TRIAZOLAM

Like alprazolam, triazolam belongs to the group of BDZs referred to as the 1,4-triazolo BDZs. The triazolo ring and the attached methyl group are responsible for the rapid oxidation by liver enzymes, resulting in a short elimination half-life and conversion to readily-excreted derivatives.

Triazolam is promptly absorbed after an oral dose, yielding peak plasma concentration (range of 2 to 10 μg/l) within 2 hours. Approximately 85% of the oral dose is absorbed in fasting subjects (Eberts et al., 1981). Peak triazolam levels seem to be higher (8.3 versus 4.0 μg/l) and occur earlier (0.8 versus 2.1 hours) in elderly than in young women. This difference does not appear in young and elderly men (Greenblatt et al., 1983). The mean Tmax after an oral dose (0.5 mg) in the evening is reported to be 2.3 hours, compared with 1.7 hours following day-time assumption (Smith et al., 1986). This suggests diurnal variations of triazolam absorption. Sublingual administration results in peak triazolam concentrations that are higher and which occur earlier than with the oral route (Kroboth et al., 1986).

Bioavailability after oral administration is approximately 61%. Around 25% of the dose of triazolam is presystemically metabolized in the liver. The apparent volume of distribution is 1.0 l/Kg irrespective of age and gender (Smith et al., 1983). Triazolam is 89% bound to human serum proteins as calculated in binding studies carried out in vitro. By using equilibrium dialysis in vivo, however, triazolam appears to be only 10-25% bound to plasma proteins. Only half is bound to albumin with the other portion bound to acid glycoprotein (Kroboth et al., 1984).

Triazolam would be expected to cross readily into the brain because of its high lipid solubility (Greenblatt et al., 1983). [^{14}C]-triazolam studies in monkeys have demonstrated high levels of radioactivity in the brain 1 hour after an oral dose of 0.5 mg/kg (Kitagawa et al., 1979). Data concerning transplacentar transfer of triazolam or its passage into breast milk in human are not available. It is able to cross the placenta in pregnant rats and it is excreted into the milk of lactating rats at a 70% concentration in material plasma (Kitagawa et al., 1979). This study suggests similar results would be seen in humans.

Triazolam undergoes hydroxylation and subsequent conjugation with glucuronic acid. The major derivative is alpha-hydroxy triazolam. The ratio of unconjugated to conjugated triazolam peak levels is almost 19%, showing that this major metabolite undergoes rapid conjugation. The plasma peak levels for alpha-hydroxy triazolam-glucuronide conjugate range from 2.7 to 10.3 μg/l (mean 6.1 μg/l) after an oral dose of 1 mg. Although alpha-hydroxy triazolam is believed to possess strong pharmacological activity, its prompt glucuronide conjugation prevents it from participating in triazolam's activity. 4-hydroxy triazolam is also detected in the plasma, along with α-hydroxy triazolam and the coniugated form of both (Sethy and Harris, 1982).

The mean elimination half life of triazolam has been quoted as between 2.3 and 3.8 hours, while the mean elimination half-life of the conjugated metabolites is shorter. Its total clearance ranges from 6.2 to 8.6 ml/min/Kg in healthy volunteers. Therefore, accumulation of triazolam or its metabolites after multiple doses does not occur (Friedman et al., 1986).

The pharmacokinetics of oral triazolam are little altered in patients with renal failure (Kroboth et al., 1985). Mild liver illnesses do not affect its hepatic metabolism. In cirrhotic patients however, the mean elimination half-life appears to be slower and the total body clearance decreased (Kroboth et al., 1987). In this case, decreasing doses are recommended.

Bibliography

Eberts FS, Pilopoulos Y, Reineke LM and Vliek RW: Triazolam disposition. *Clinical Pharmacology and Therapeutics* 29:81-93, 1981

Friedman H, Greenblatt DJ, Burnstein ES, Harvatz JS and Shader RI: Population study of triazolam pharmacokinetics. *British Journal of Clinical Pharmacology* 22:639-642, 1986

Greenblatt DJ, Arendt RM, Abernethy DR, Giles HG, Sellers EM, et al.: In vitro quantification of benzodiazepine lipophilicity: relation to in vivo distribution. *British Journal of Anaesthesiology* 55:985-989, 1983

Greenblatt DJ, Divoll M, Abernethy DR, Moschitto LJ, Smith RB, et al.: Reduced clearance of triazolam in old age: relation to antipyrine oxidizing capacity. *British Journal of Clinical Pharmacology* 15:303-309, 1983

Kitagawa H, Esumi Y, Krurosawa S, Sekine S and Yokoshima T: Metabolism of 8-chloro-6-(ochlorophenyl)-1-methyl-4H-s-triazolo (4,3a) (1,4) benzodiazepine, triazolam, a new central depressant, I: absorption, distribution and excretion in rats, dogs, and monkeys. *Xenobiotica* 9:415-428, 1979

Kroboth PD, Smith RB, Rosanske T, Hamilton JM, McAuley JW, et al.: Triazolam route of administration studies, I: pharmacokinetics. *Abstract Pharmaceutical Research* 3(S):111, 1986

Kroboth PD, Smith RB, Silver MR, Rault R, Sorkin MI, et al.: Effects of end stage renal disease and aluminium hydroxide on triazolam pharmacokinetics. *British Journal of Clinical Pharmacology* 27:555-560, 1985

Kroboth PD, Smith RB, Sorkin MI, Silver M, Rault R, et al.: Triazolam protein binding correlation with alpha-1 acid glycoprotein concentration. *Clinical Pharmacology and Therapeutics* 36:379-383, 1984

Kroboth PD, Smith RB, Van Thiel DH and Juhl RP: Night-time dosing of triazolam in patients with liver disease and normal subjects: kinetics and daytime effects. *Journal of Clinical Pharmacology* 27:555-560, 1987

Sethy VH and Harris DW: Determination of biological activity of alprazolam, triazolam and their metabolites. *Journal of Pharmacy and Pharmacology* 34:115-116, 1982

Smith RB, Divoll M, Gillespie WR and Greenblatt DJ: Effect of subject age and gender on the pharmacokinetics of oral triazolam and temazepam. *Journal of Clinical Psychopharmacology* 3:172-176, 1983

Smith RB, Kroboth PD and Phillips JP: Temporal variation in triazolam pharmacokinetics and pharmacodynamics after oral administration. *Journal of Clinical Pharmacology* 26:120-124,1986

Benzodiazepine Side Effects

Central effects

The most common side effect of BDZs is the depressogenic effect on the CNS, which mainly manifests in the form of sedation, myorelaxation and amnesia (Hobbs et al., 1996).

BDZs given for antianxiety therapy should not produce a generalized sedation. The degree of sedation, which may be higher in elderly patients, can cause problems to patients for example at work or when driving (Linnoila and Ellinwood, 1983). An excessive depression of the CNS may occur clinically to create several effects: myasthenia, ataxia, dysartria, diplopia, blurred vision, apathy, vertigo, confusion or drowsiness (Finkle, 1983; Lemerc, 1960).

CNS depression is almost constantly dose-dependent, since it occurs more often in patients who take high doses and are more susceptible, unlike patients whose anamnesis includes a history of alcohol or barbiturate abuse. Another observation points out that there is a lower occurrence of drowsiness among smokers than non-smokers. More infrequently, BDZs may produce stimulation rather than sedation (paradoxical effect) in some subjects. It is not clear whether all BDZs have the potential ability to induce these effects, which have been observed with diazepam, chlordiazepoxide, clorazepam and oxazepam.

Clinically, a state of excitation was noticed with signs of clear hostility and excessive irritability. Some authors interpret this appearance of hostility as a behavioural response to the pharmacologically induced reduction of anxiety, and have suggested (Priest et al., 1980) the existence of a mechanism of action analogous to the disinhibiting effect of BDZs in animal behaviour.

In the case of the parenteral use of BDZs — particularly when they are rapidly infused intravenously — cases of acute cardiovascular and respiratory depressions are reported, with hypotension or apnoea (Doughty, 1970). Epidemiological data are not available to explain this phenomenon precisely. But the existence of serious concomitant diseases and/or the concurrent use of other CNS-depressant drugs in these cases requires some caution in using this type of administration, and makes its use advisable only in patients specifically requiring it.

Peripheral effects

- Hepatotoxicity: studies on hepatic functionality during different treatments with BDZs have not provided evidence of substantial changes which may be ascribed to these medications.
- Although some hematic changes induced by BDZs have occurred on occasion, this is nevertheless an extremely infrequent event; in non cases, the pancytopenia and a granulocytosis observed might be definitely ascribed to the effect of these medications only.
- Allergic reactions: allergic dermatites in the form of urticaria, maculopapular eruptions, angioneurotic edema may arise during treatment with chlordiazepoxide; photosensistivity-induced reactions have also occurred, as well as swelling of the tongue.

Bibliography

Doughty A: Unexpected danger of diazepam. *British Medical Journa*l 2:239, 1970.

Finkle BS: Benzodiazepine overdosage. In: *Pharmacology of benzodiazepines.* Usdin E, Skolnick P, Tallman JF, Greenblatt D and Paul SM (eds.) Verlag Chemie, Weinheim, pp. 619-628, 1983

Hobbs WR, Rall TW and Verdoorn TA: Hypnotics and sedatives; ethanol. In: *Goodman and Gilman's the pharmacological basis of therapeutics.* Hardman JG, Limbird LE, Molinoff PB, Ruddon RW and Goodman Gilman A (eds.). 9th Edition McGraw-Hill, New York pp. 361-396, 1996

Lemerc F: Toxic reactions to chlordiazeposside. *Journal of American Medical Association* 174: 893, 1960

Linnoila M and Ellinwood E: Effects of benzodiazepines on performance of healthy volunteers and anxious and elderly patients In: *Pharmacology of benzodiazepines*. Usdin E, Skolnick P, Tallman JF, Greenblatt D and Paul SM (eds.), Verlag Chemie, Weinheim, pp. 601-608, 1983

Priest RG, Vianna Filho U, Amrein R and Skreta M: *Benzodiazepines today and tomorrow*. MTP Press Limited, Lancaster, England, 1980.

Priest RG: The Benzodiazepines. A clinical review. In: *Benzodiazepines today and tomorrow*. Priest RG, Vianna Filho U, Amrein R and Skreta M (eds.), MTP Press Limited, Lancaster, pp. 77-83, 1980.

Benzodiazepine Toxicity

Toxic effects

BDZs are used extensively all over the world as sedative-hypnotic and antianxiety drugs. An unavoidable consequence of this is that they are becoming more and more involved in cases of intoxication, either intentional with self-destructive intent or accidental.

The evaluation of this subject, both from a social and a medical point of view, is a matter of strong and differing opinions. On the one hand, it is argued that the level of BDZs' clinical toxicity is very low, and therefore cannot induce serious or fatal intoxications (Matthew, 1974; Davis et al., 1968). Others however, suggest that these drugs may cause death in cases of overdosages (Barraclough, 1974). According to statistics, the incidence of cases of poisoning connected with BDZ derivatives varies in time and depending on locations, with values ranging between 20% and 50% (Greenblatt et al., 1977).

It should be pointed out that cases of poisoning induced by more than one drug occur more frequently than cases where a single drug is involved. The rather obvious explanation for this fact is that patients at risk from self-destructive actions have different kinds of drugs at their disposal, and also that alcohol is available everywhere. The association of BDZs plus barbiturates represents a very dangerous combination for such patients who, in these cases, reach a central nervous system depression up to the 4th degree, some even requiring respiratory assistance. It is therefore advisable to make a distinction between the consequences of intoxication induced by BDZs only and intoxication resulting from BDZs taken concurrently with other types of drugs (Finkle, 1983; Mattew et al., 1972).

In the case of intoxication caused by BDZs alone, the clinical signs do not appear to go beyond a state of torpor, which may be more or less deep depending on the ingested doses, with concomitant ataxia and dysarthria. Hypotension and respiratory insufficiency may occur, although infrequently. Attempts have been made to determine the "lethal" doses of BDZs. With chlordiazepoxide for instance, it was noticed that plasma levels exceeding 20 μg/ml are associated with states of coma up to the third degree: but, "comas depassés" were never observed even with levels exceeding 60 μg/ml. However, it should be considered that therapeutic doses of this medication produce concentrations in plasma of up to 30 μg/l (Greenblatt and Shader, 1974).

Teratogenic effects

The teratogenic effects of BDZs or the toxic effects of these medications on the fetus is a controversial question. Conclusive evaluations of a group of epidemiological studies (Milkovich and Van der Berg, 1974; Martz et al., 1985; Morselli, 1977; Goldberg and DiMascio, 1978) indicate that a non-causal relationship exists in man between BDZs and congenital defects (Hines, 1981). A small increase in the risk of midline cleft deformities of the lip or palate is the most persistent, but there has also been the suggestion — not yet proven — of a relationship between BDZs and congenital defects (Safra and Oakley, 1975).

The depressogenic effect of BDZs on the CNS may be present in the neonate, and especially in the premature newborn. Regarding the use of anxiolytics by nursing women, who might transmit these substances to the neonate through their milk, thus involving some possible adverse effects, it has been shown that small amounts of the medication have been found in milk for diazepam, chlordiazepoxide, oxazepam and clordiazepate (Hines, 1981). Some defects could also be noticed in the newborn, EEG changes and lethargy occurring after high doses had been taken. The fetus and the newborn have a lower capacity to metabolize BDZs than adults.

Bibliography

Barraclough BM: Are there safer hypnotic than barbiturates? Lancet 1:57-58, 1974.

Davis JM, Barlett E and Termini BA: Overdosage of psychotropic drugs: a review. *Dis Nervous System* 29:157-164, 1968

Finkle BS: Benzodiazepine overdosage In: Pharmacology of benzodiazepines. Usdin E, Skolnick P, Tallman JF, Greenblatt Dand Paul SM (eds.) *Verlag Chemie, Weinheim,* pp. 619-628, 1983

Goldberg HL and DiMascio A: Psychotropic drugs in pregnancy. In: *Psychopharmacology: a generation of progress.* Lipton MA, DiMascio A and Killam KF (eds.), Raven Press, New York, pp. 1047-1055, 1978

Greenblatt DJ, Allen MD, Noel BJ and Shader RI: Acute overdosage with benzodiazepines derivatives. *Clinical Pharmacology and Therapeutics* 21: 497-514, 1977

Greenblatt DJ and Shader RI: Benzodiazepines. *New England Journal of Medicine* 291:1239-1243, 1974

Greenblatt DJ and Shader RI: *Benzodiazepines in clinical practice.* Raven Press, New York, 242-253, 1974
Hines LR: Toxicology and side-effects of anxiolytics. In: *Psychotropic agents. Handbook of experimental pharmacology.* Hoffmeister F and Stille G. (eds.), Springer-Verlag, Berlin 55/II pp. 359-393, 1981
Martz SC, Meinone OP, Shapiro S, Siskind V and Slone D: Antenatal exposure to meprobamate and chlordiazepesside in relation to malformations, mental development and childhood mortality. *New England Journal of Medicine* 292:726-728, 1975
Matthew M, Prondfoot AT, Brown SS and Aitken RCB: Acute poisoning. A comparison of hypnotic drugs. *Practitioner* 208:254-258, 1972
Matthew M: Are there safer hypnotics than barbiturates? *Lancet* 1:224, 1974
Milkovich L and Van der Berg BJ: Effects of prenatal meprobamate and chlordiazeposside hydrochloride on human embryonic and fetal development. *New England Journal of Medicine* 291:1268-1271, 1974
Morselli PL: Psychotropic drugs. In: *Drug disposition during development.* Morselli PL (ed.) Spectrum Publications, Inc. New York, pp. 431-474, 1977
Safra MJ and Oakley GP: Association between cleft lip with or without cleft palate and prenatal exposure to diazepam. *Lancet* 2:478-480, 1975

Dependence and Tolerance

Since BDZs were introduced in the 1960s, their use has increased to the extent that according to some estimates, at least 2% of the adult population has taken a BDZ daily for at least a six month period (Mellinger et al., 1984). The trend of rising consumption of BDZs has recently abated, mainly due to concerns over the potential hazards related to long term treatment. Even so, although antianxiety medications have never been introduced in human therapy, an extensive use of BDZs still predominates. The reason that BDZ anxiolytics are so widely used is that they are still considered extremely effective drugs, safe and devoid of dependence-inducing properties. However, recent evidence questions these assumptions and raises concerns related to the safety, efficacy and advisability of prolonged treatments with BDZs (American Psychiatric Association, 1990). The future role of BDZs in anxiolytic therapy depends strictly on the contentious issues of tolerance, withdrawal and dependence. In view of the considerable clinical implications of these problems, it is essential they are correctly understood, and managed by the prescribing physician in order to preserve an important class of anti-anxiety medicines and to recommend their appropriate use.

The administration of BDZs has been reported to produce tolerance to their pharmacological effects both in animals and in humans, so that, in some cases, their efficacy is substantially hindered by tolerance (Higgitt et al., 1988).

Acute tolerance appears when, after a single dose, the pharmacological effects of a given BDZ plasma concentration decline once the omega modulatory sites have been exposed to the drug over even a short period. Therefore, a given BDZ plasma concentration may be able to induce a certain action during the absorption phase (when the plasma levels are increasing), whereas the same plasma concentration may lack any effect a few hours later, during the distribution phase (when the plasma levels are decreasing).

The concept of the minimal effective plasma concentration is a useful parameter in terms of a theoretical pharmacokinetics. The results are no longer indicative of the actual duration of action of a given BDZ, because some pharmacological effects may be attenuated by the development of the pharmacodynamic tolerance, sooner than expected on the basis of a purely pharmacokinetic model.

The extent and rate of development of acute tolerance are different among the various BDZ compounds. After single doses, alprazolam and lorazepam, two BDZ agents with similar half-life elimination show a different development of acute tolerance to cognitive impairment, the pharmacological effects lasting much less with the former compound. Moreover, a single dose of a given BDZ induces several pharmacological actions, and tolerance to each one may develop at different rate. The duration of these actions is further affected by chronic tolerance induced by repetitive dosing (Greenblatt and Shader, 1986). Chronic tolerance develops when, after repeated administrations, a given dose of BDZ produces a reduced effect and an increasingly larger dose must be administered to obtain the effects observed with the original dose. Chronic tolerance has been demonstrated to most of the behavioural effects of BDZs in animals, and it develops at different rates for different actions. Chronic tolerance to sedative effects can be observed after two or three days, to anticonvulsant actions after four days and anxiolytic effects after two or three weeks. Conversely, evidence suggests that chronic tolerance to the locomotor stimulant responses of low doses of BDZ does not occur. This differential rate of development of tolerance to the various behavioural effects of BDZs supports the hypothesis that the phenomenon is mediated by different biochemical mechanisms (Haigh and Feely, 1988; File, 1985).

In human pharmacology, chronic tolerance develops to the sedative effects of BDZs. Thus, most patients with initial drowsiness report that it declines within a few days, despite continued dosing and increasing plasma levels. Also, the degree and rate of development of chronic tolerance differ among the various BDZ derivatives. For example, lorazepam is reported to be associated with the development of more tolerance than either the long-acting agent, ketazolam, or the short-acting compound, triazolam. In addition, tolerance to lorazepam appears more rapidly then tolerance to oxazepam, despite the very similar pharmacokinetic profiles. The sedative, anticonvulsant and performance-impairing effects of most BDZ compounds are widely affected by chronic tolerance, and therefore are weakly correlated with plasma concentrations. Whether tolerance to the antianxiety effects also develops is still controversial. The BDZs are undoubtedly effective anxiolytics in the short term, but whether or not they maintain their clinical efficacy upon chronic administration has not been effectively demonstrated in controlled trials. Clinical experience suggests that they do remain therapeutically beneficial. In fact, the anxiolytic effect of BDZs seems to plateau, as expected, according to drug plasma concentration, since this effect does not appear to be subject to much chronic tolerance. Therefore, since different clinical effects have different courses of tolerance, this makes it difficult to establish the "duration of action" for a given BDZ, as it depends on which clinical action is being evaluated and how the duration is measured (Lader and File, 1987).

Tolerance to anxiolytic effects does not commonly occur with the BDZs in terms of requiring increasing doses. The need for continued medication reflects more the necessity to prevent withdrawal than to maintain efficacy. Since patients seeking treatments for anxiety or insomnia typically have chronic conditions and BDZs reduce these disorders, recurrence of the symptomatology for which the medication was originally taken should be expected after the drug is discontinued. Symptom recurrence generally occurs slowly, over a period of weeks or months, after stopping treatment. It is similar in character to premorbid symptomatology, and should be no more severe in intensity than the original symptoms. Alternatively, symptoms of the original disorder may occur in an intensity greater than experienced at the start of therapy. This excessive recurrence of symptoms is termed rebound. Rebound symptomatology usually develops within hours to days of BDZs' discontinuation, with a precise time course, partly depending on the pharmacokinetic properties of the particular compound. Recurrence and rebound result from the relapse of the underlying disorder that preceded treatment.

The BDZ withdrawal syndrome differs qualitatively from either recurrence or rebound in that it has an important autonomic component. It is now a well established fact that most BDZs produce physical dependence after prolonged treatment, which is demonstrated by the occurrence of withdrawal symptoms upon abrupt or gradual discontinuation of medication. Although psychiatrists previously felt that patients could become dependent on BDZs only after long term therapy in high dosages, it is well known that some degree of dependence can develop after only a few days of treatment with BDZ hypnotics, or after four-six weeks therapy with BDZ anxiolytics. As a result, symptoms may occur after only a short duration of treatment. Prominent symptoms include excess sensitivity to light and sound, insomnia, tachycardia, mild systolic hypertension, tremulously, sweating, abdominal distress, headache, dysphoria, depersonalization and lethargy (Greenblatt et al., 1990).

The withdrawal syndrome may supervene despite carefully tapering the dose, and become evident 2-10 days after stopping the treatment. Like rebound, the withdrawal syndrome is self-limited and patients should recover completely if it occurs.

Daily BDZ dose, length of therapy, half-life and drug potency all contribute to the patient's difficulty, which is experienced when attempting to discontinue chronic BDZ intake. In addition, initial psychopathology level, diagnosis and personality also contribute to withdrawal severity.

Withdrawal symptoms are easily treated. The BDZ can either be restarted and then slowly withdrawn or substituted by another BDZ with a longer half-life, given on a short term basis, which is then gradually withdrawn. The use of phenothiazines or tricyclis to treat withdrawal symptoms is contraindicated, since they lower the seizure threshold thereby increasing the risk of convulsion (Dupont, 1990).

Rebound, withdrawal and the development of tolerance to certain pharmacodynamic effects suggest the action of some compensatory mechanism to antagonize the effect of the drug.

It is possible to assume that an equilibrium is reached between the effects of the drug and the compensatory neurobiological mechanisms. When this equilibrium is disrupted by stopping the drug abruptly, there may be rebound and/or withdrawal symptoms as the compensatory mechanisms persist because they are not antagonized. The symptoms last until the induced compensatory mechanism can return to the baseline state with gradual cessation of the drug. These adaptive mechanisms have the opportunity to readjust in step with reducing quantities of the drug, reducing or avoiding rebound symptoms.

The neurochemical mechanisms underlying tolerance, dependence and withdrawal are not yet fully understood. They require receptor occupation since co-administration of the BDZ receptor antagonist, flumazenil, or inverse agonist, CGS8216, can prevent the development of tolerance (File, 1982; Eisenberg, 1987). The view that tolerance and withdrawal are receptor-related events is supported by the evidence that:

- withdrawal symptomatology may be precipitated by a rapid displacement of the agonist from the receptor by using the antagonist
- full agonists induce more severe tolerance than partial agonists (Haigh and Feely, 1988).

A number of investigations have attempted to determine whether changes in BDZ receptor number and affinity were implicated in the pathogenesis of tolerance and withdrawal.

The behavioural tolerance manifestations appear to be associated with biochemical alterations indicative of receptor down regulation, including decreased BDZ binding and reduced efficacy of GABA/muscimol-stimulated chloride flux (Miller et al., 1988; Miller et al., 1989b).

Conversely, chronic administration of either the BDZ antagonist flumazenil, or the partial inverse agonist F6-7142 has been shown to produce neurochemical changes, which suggest an up regulation of the BDZ receptor complex expressed by an increase in the number of BDZ sites and in the maximum muscimol-stimulated chloride uptake (Miller et al., 1989a; Pritchard et al., 1991).

These data indicate that tolerance to BDZs might involve not only the omega modulatory site, but also overall function at the GABA receptor. It is likely that prolonged administration alters the receptor's configuration, perhaps leading to decreased coupling between GABA and the chloride channel (Marley and Gallenger, 1989).

A possible locus of receptor modulation may be GABA receptor gene expression. However, recent studies using lorazepam show that mRNA for the $alpha_1$, and $gamma_2$ subunits is decreased during chronic administration, but this change occurs subsequent to the development of tolerance and receptor down regulation (Kang and Miller, 1991).

Chronic BDZ administration might also have post-translational effects, perhaps altering desensitization, or altering the receptor half-life, which occurs in the other neurotransmitter systems (Gallager et al., 1984).

One interesting theory regarding withdrawal is that the continued administration of BDZ agonists and inverse agonists is associated with a change in receptor-ionophore coupling (Nutt, 1990). The effect, described as a "withdrawal shift", is an increase in the intrinsic properties of inverse agonists and a decrease in the properties of agonists. According to this hypothesis, the changes appear without alterations in receptor number or affinity, and may reflect a shift in efficacy at the receptor.

It has been reported that treatment with flumazenil during BDZ agonist administration, or even in the period after the last dose, could prevent or reverse this efficacy shift, as indicated by a lack of sensitization to inverse agonists (Nutt and Castello, 1988). However, conflicting results have been reported on this topic, and further observations are required to confirm this point (Cittadini and Lader, 1991).

Preliminary results suggest that when acting on the BDZ modulatory site, the newer anxiolytic non BDZ compounds, such as cyclopyrrolones and imidazolopyridine, fail to produce a receptor shift, despite being full agonists. They also seem to possess less propensity to induce tolerance and dependence upon prolonged administration (Morton and Lader, 1990; Schoch et al., 1991).

Bibliography

American Psychiatric Association: Benzodiazepine dependence, toxicity and abuse. *Task Force Report*, Washington, DC, 1990

Cittadini A and Lader M: Lack of effect of a small dose of flumazenil in reversing short-term tolerance to benzodiazepine in normal subjects. *Psychopharmacology* 5:220-227, 1991

Dupont RL: A practical approach to benzodiazepine discontinuation. *Journal of Psychiatric Research* 24:8190, 1990

Eisenberg RM: Diazepam withdrawal as demonstrated by changes in plasma corticosterone: a role for the hippocampus. *Life Sciences* 40:817-825, 1987

File SE: Tolerance to the behavioural action of benzodiazepines. *Neuroscience Bio Behaviour Reviews* 9:113-122, 1985

File SE: Recovery from lorazepam tolerance and the effects of a benzodiazepine antagonist (RO 15-1788) on the development of tolerance. *Psychopharmacology* 77:284, 1982

Gallager DW, Lakoski JM, Gonsalves SF and Ranch SC: Chronic benzodiazepine treatment decreases postsynaptic GABA sensitivity. *Nature* 290:514-516, 1984

Greenblatt DJ, Miller LG and Shader RI: Benzodiazepine discontinuation syndromes. *Journal of Psychiatric Research* 24 (suppl 2):73-79, 1990

Greenblatt DJ and Shader RI: Long-term administration of benzodiazepines: pharmacokinetic versus pharmacodynamic tolerance. *Psychopharmacology Bulletin* 22:416-423, 1986

Haigh JRM and Feely M: Tolerance to the anticonvulsant effect of benzodiazepines. *Trends Pharmacological Sciences* 9: 361-366, 1988

Higgitt A, Fonegy P and Lader M: The natural history of tolerance to the benzodiazepines. *Psychol Med Monograph Suppl. 13* Cambridge, Cambridge University Press, 1988

Kang I and Miller LG: Decreased $GABA_A$ receptor subunit mRNA concentrations following chronic lorazepam administration. *British Journal of Pharmacology*, 103: 1285-1287, 1991

Lader MH and File S: The biological basis for benzodiazepine dependence. *Psychological Medicine* 17:539, 1987

Marley RJ and Gallenger DW: Chronic diazepam treatment produces regionally specific changes in GABAstimulated chloride influx. *European Journal of Pharmacology* 159:217-223, 1989

Mellinger GD, Balter MB and Uhlnhoth EH: Prevalence and correlates of long term use of benzodiazepine. *Journal of American Medical Association* 251:375-379, 1984

Miller LG, Greenblatt DJ, Barnhill JG and Shader RI: Benzodiazepine administration I tolerance is associated with BDZ receptor downregulation and decreased $GABA_A$ receptor function. *Journal of Pharmacology and Experimental Therapeutics* 246:170-176, 1988

Miller LG, Greenblatt DJ, Roy RB, Gaver A, Lopez F and Shader RI: Chronic benzodiazepine administration. III. Upregulation of gamma-aminobutyric $acid_A$ receptor binding and function associated with chronic benzodiazepine antagonist administration. *Journal of Pharmacology and Experimental Therapeutics* 248:1096-1101, 1989a

Miller LG, Woolverton S, Greemlatt DS, Lopez F, Roy RB and Shader RI: Chronic benzodiazepine administration IV rapid development of tolerance and receptor downregulation associated with alprazolam administration. *Biochemical Pharmacology* 38:3773-3777, 1989b

Morton S and Lader M: Studies with alpidem in normal volunteers and anxious patients. *Pharmacopsychiatry* 23:120, 1990

Nutt DJ: Pharmacological mechanisms of benzodiazepine withdrawal. *Journal of Psychological Research 24* (suppl. 2):105-110, 1990

Nutt DJ and Castello M: Rapid induction of lorazepam dependence and its reversal with flumazenil. *Life Sciences* 43:1045-1053, 1988

Pritchard GA, Galfen WR, Lumpkin M and Miller LG: Chronic benzodiazepine administration VIII receptor upregulation produced by chronic exposure to the inverse agonist FG-7142. *Journal of Pharmacology and Experimental Therapeutics* 258:280-285, 1991

Schoch P, Facklam M and Haefely WE: Comparative pharmacology of full and partial agonists at the benzodiazepine receptor. *European Neuropsychopharmacology* 1 (3):185-486, 1991

Benzodiazepine Interactions

It is necessary to study interactions between medications since the concurrent administration of two substances may enhance or decrease the expected effect, as well as give rise on occasion to unwanted actions. BDZs strongly enhance the effects of alcohol, barbiturates and all other central nervous system depressants (Hobbs et al., 1996).

The solution of diazepam used for intravenous injections contains propylene glycol, and this increases the depressant and hypotensive properties of the compound.

Although BDZs have a high binding rate with plasma proteins, no interaction through displacement induced by other medications such as sulfamides, minor analgesics and oral coagulants has been observed. Other cases of interaction exist, although their cause is still unknown:

a — phenytoin associated with BDZs reaches higher plasma levels, with increased toxicity.

b — BDZs produce ecchymoses in patients who make chronic use of oral anticoagulants.

c — if administered with levodopa, they increase tremor in subjects affected by Parkinsons disease.

d — side effects are less frequent in heavy smokers than in non smokers, since smoke induces the synthesis of hepatic catabolic enzymes.

e — the concomitant use with antidepressants produces a depressant effect on the central nervous system (drowsiness, loss of memory, impairment of motor performance).

f — with decamethonium and curare, they potentiate the effect of neuromuscular block.
g — with hydantoinic antiepileptics, the effect is enhanced.
h — valproic acid associated with BDZs may precipitate psychotic episodes.

Bibliography

Hobbs WR, Rall TW and Verdoorn TA: Hypnotics and sedatives; ethanol. In: *Goodman and Gilman's the pharmacological basis of therapeutics.* Hardman JG, Limbird LE, Molinoff PB, Ruddon RW and Goodman Gilman A (eds.). 9th Edition McGraw-Hill, New York pp. 361-396, 1996

GABAergic System in the Action of Anxiolytic Drugs

The presence of GABA in the mammalian CNS was discovered around 1950 (Roberts and Frankel, 1950) and few years later its function, as an inhibitory neurotransmitter, was identified. Today, GABA is the most known amino acid neurotransmitter playing an inhibitory role in the CNS. Many GABAergic pathways have been identified in the CNS and their important role in the control of behavioral and endocrine functions in physiological and pathological conditions is under investigation (Enna, 1984; Racagni and Donoso, 1986; Biggio and Costa, 1990).

Almost all the GABA present in the brain — where it is distributed discretely — originates from glutamic acid. Indeed GABA metabolism is intimately related to the glutamate and glutamine cycles. The alpha-decarboxylation of glutamic acid into GABA is catalyzed by glutamic acid decarboxylase (GAD), an enzyme that occurs almost uniquely in the mammalian CNS and retinal tissue. In general, the precise localization of GAD in the brain correlates quite well with GABA content. The enzyme GABA aminotransferase (GABA-T), responsible for GABA transamination into succinic semialdehyde, is widely distributed in the brain. Succinic semialdehyde is then rapidly oxidized by succinic semialdehyde dehydrogenase to succinic acid, which reenters the Krebs cycle (De Robertis, 1986).

A significant amount of GABA is stored in the nerve terminals, and following depolarization, released in the intersynaptic cleft. At this level, GABA interacts with specific GABA receptors or is taken up, by an active transport process, into the nerve terminals and glial cells (figure 1, page 63).

Two types of GABA receptors, called $GABA_A$ and $GABA_B$, have been discovered. $GABA_A$ receptors (as will be discussed extensively) are the tar-

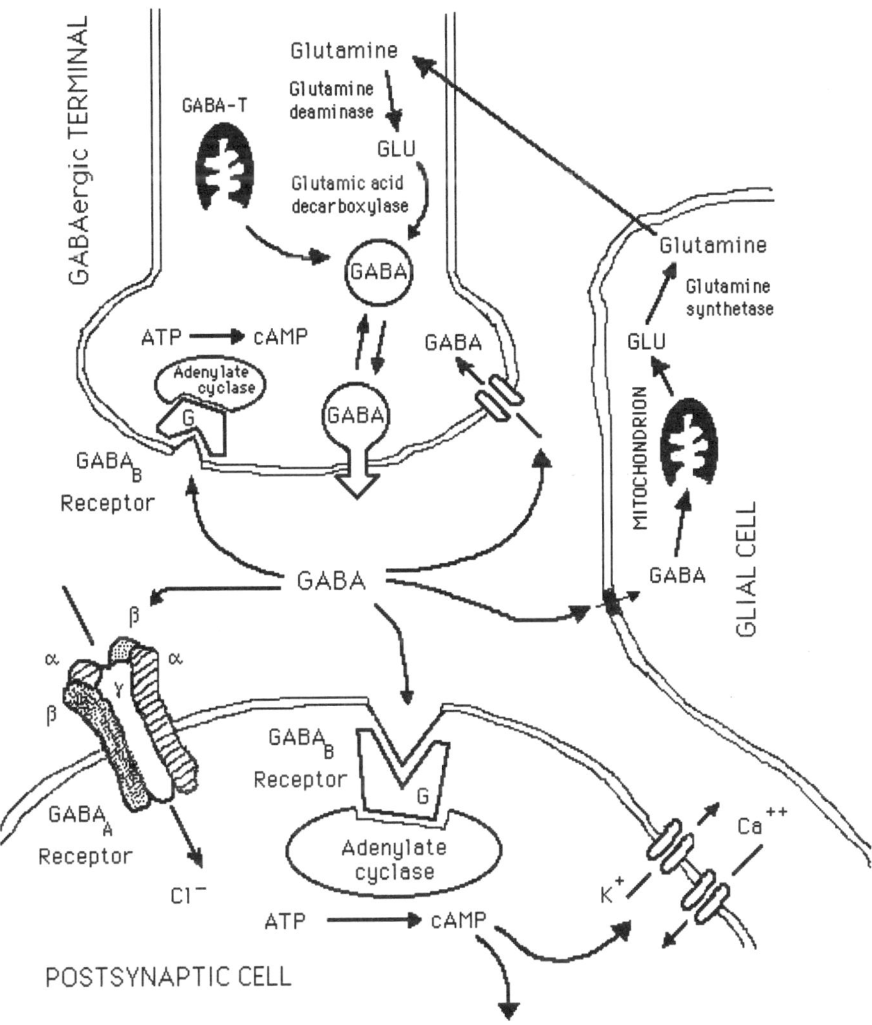

Fig. 1: Schematic representation of a GABAergic synapse. The major pathways for the synthesis and degradation of GABA are also shown. GABA uptake by the terminal and the glial cell serve as the primary mechanism for terminating the action of GABA in the intersynaptic cleft. Activation of GABA$_A$ receptors causes an opening of the ion channel and triggers a Cl$^-$ in-flow into the cell with consequent hyperpolarization of the neuron. GABA$_B$ receptors are linked to adenylate cyclase enzyme. GABA$_B$ receptors present on nerve terminal appear to inhibit neurotransmitter release. ATP, adenosine triphosphate; cAMP, cyclic adenosine monophosphate; G, G protein; GABA-T, GABA aminotransferase.

get of BDZs and other anxiolytic drugs. BDZ activation of $GABA_A$ receptors in specific CNS areas is also responsible for other pharmacological effects, such as anticonvulsant, sedative and sleep potentiation (table 3, page 65).

Activating the $GABA_B$ receptors, which are mainly located on the axon terminals of non GABAergic neurons, modifies the neurotransmitter release from these neurons. Stimulating the $GABA_B$ receptors induces a miorelaxant effect. Baclofen, a specific $GABA_B$ agonist, has been used for a number of years to treat spasticity (Bowery et al., 1990).

Bibliography

Biggio G and Costa E: *GABA and benzodiazepine receptor subtypes*. Raven Press, New York, 1990

Bowery NG, Knott C, Moratalla R and Pratt GD: $GABA_B$ receptors and their heterogeneity. In: *GABA and benzodiazepine receptor subtypes*. Biggio G and Costa E (eds.) Raven Press, New York, pp. 127-139, 1990

De Robertis E: GABAergic neurotransmission. An overview. In: *GABA and endocrine function*. Racagni G and Donoso AO (eds.) Raven Press, New York, pp. 1-12, 1986

Enna SJ: *The GABA receptors*. The Humana Press, Clifton, NJ, 1983

Roberts E and Frankel S: Gamma-aminobutyric acid in brain: its formation from glutamic acid. *Journal of Biological Chemistry* 187:55-63, 1950

Racagni G and Donoso AO: *GABA and endocrine function*. Raven Press, New York, 1986

GABA Receptor and Anxiolytic Drugs

The $GABA_A$ receptor is the most abundant inhibitory receptor in the mammalian brain. It has a heteropolymeric structure that forms a chloride-channel (figure 2, page 66).

The binding of the two molecules of the neurotransmitter to the specific recognition site on the $GABA_A$ receptor opens the ion channel and triggers a Cl^- in-flow into the cell, which hyperpolarizes the neuron, preventing activation by the incoming depolarizing stimuli. This Cl^- inward flow may be modulated both by endogenous substances and by drugs which operate as positive or negative allosteric regulators. GABA action may be affected by isosteric receptor antagonists, which, it has been suggested, bind to the extracellular domain of the receptor. Allosteric regulation is operated by two different classes of compounds, a) those that act on the extracellular domain and b) those that act on the channel domain of the receptor. Both classes include positive and negative allosteric modulators. The positive modulators acting on the extracellular domain include BDZs, imidazolopyridines (alpidem, zolpidem), cyclopyrrolones (zopiclone, suriclone), imidazopyridines (divaplon), triazolopyridazines (CL 218872), pyrazolopyridine (ICI 190622).

Table 3 BENZODIAZEPINE ACTIONS MEDIATED BY GABA IN THE CNS

Action	Site of Interaction	Sperimental data supporting GABA involvement	Pharmacological effect
Facilitation of presynaptic inhibition	Spinal Cord	Blocked by bicuculline, picrotoxin and thiosemicarbazide	Miorelaxant
Facilitation of presynaptic inhibition	Cuneate nucleus	Blocked by bicuculline	Athassia
Facilitation of presynaptic inhibition	Genicolate nucleus	Blocked by picrotoxin	Athassia
Dopaminergic terminals inhibition	Basal ganglia	Blocked by picrotoxin	Motor incoordination
cGMP decrease	Cerebellum	Blocked by picrotoxin	Anticonvulsant activity
Decreased electric activity of Purkinje cells	Cerebellum	Antagonized by picrotoxin and bicuculline	Anticonvulsant activity and athassia
Antagonism of isoniazide- and thiosemicarbazide-induced convulsion	Cerebral cortex	Antagonized by GABA GABA-agonists and GABA-mimetics	Anticonvulsant activity
Sleep potentiation	Reticular system and cerebral cortex	Induced by GABA-mimetics and GABA-agonists	Sedative and euipnic activity
Conflict test	Limbic and cortical system	Antagonized by picrotoxin mimecked by muscimol and GABA-agonists	Antianxiety effect

The list of the negative modulators mainly consists of beta-carboline derivatives. Positive and negative allosteric modulators that interact with the extracellular domain of the $GABA_A$ receptors are antagonized by the imidazobenzodiazepinone, flumazenil. On the other hand, drugs which bind within the channel domain can act as both positive (barbiturates and steroid hormone derivatives) or negative (pregnenolone sulphate and picrotoxin) allosteric modulators (figure 2).

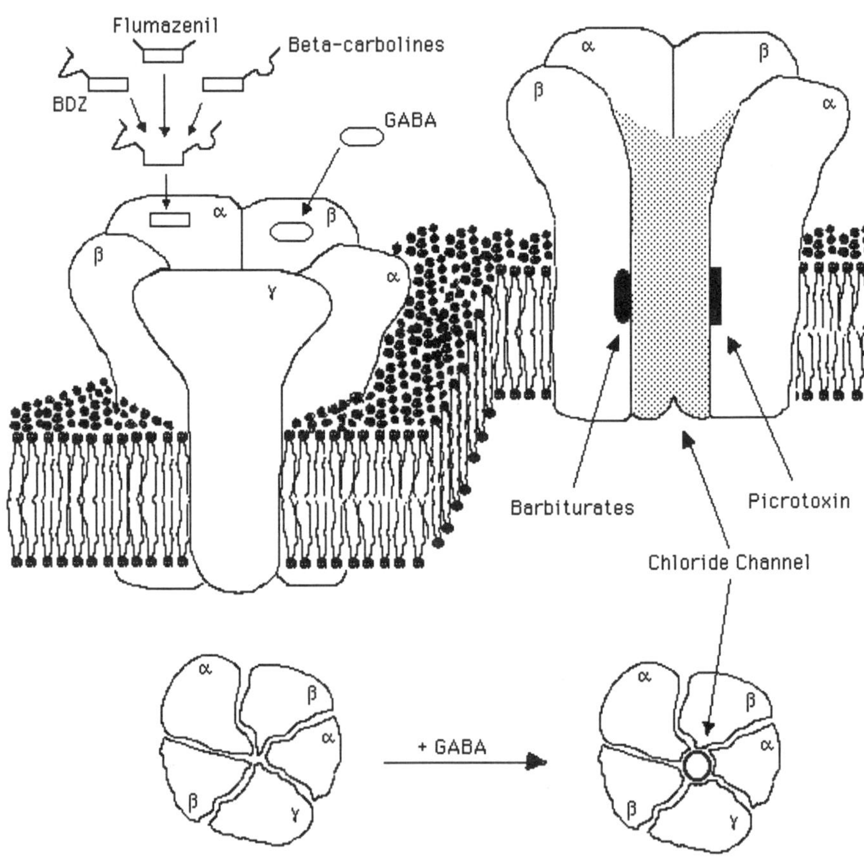

Fig. 2: Schematic representation of the $GABA_A$ macromolecular receptor complex.

The $GABA_A$ receptor belongs to the superfamily of ligand-gated ion channels, and is constructed by several homologous subunits to form the Cl^-

conducting pore. The receptor is an integral part of one or several subunits of a transmembrane hetero-oligomeric glycoprotein complex. Determining the molecular size of the intact receptor suggests it is assembled from four sub-units: however, a model with a pentameric structure is required to adapt an estimated open channel diameter of 6 Amstrong. This predicted structural feature is shared with nicotic and glycine receptors, but differs from G protein coupled receptors. The structural similarities within the superfamily of ligand gated receptors have led to the hypothesis that they evolve from a common ancestral predecessor. Two subunits of the $GABA_A$ receptor (alpha and beta) were cloned in 1987 (Schofield et al., 1987). Since then, several additional subunits (gamma, delta, epsilon, rho) and subunit variants have been cloned, bringing the total number of identified subunits to 15. The transfection of eukaryotic cell lines with a cDNA encoding various GABA receptor subunits makes possible to investigate the biophysical and pharmacological nature of every possible subtype of GABA receptor. Molecular cloning investigations have recently revealed the primary structures of the subunits proposed to constitute the sopramolecular complex of the $GABA_A$ receptor channel. All subunit classes share 35-45% sequence identity and the variants within each class display more than 70% identity. Co-expression studies, using cloned subunit variants in mammalian cells, have given rise to subunit combinations that respond to GABA — the responses can be modulated by BDZs. Recent research has provided evidence that transfected cells expressing only alpha and beta subunits form GABA gated chloride channels which weakly respond to GABA — whereas they can be antagonized by bicuculline and picrotoxin or facilitated by barbiturates. They are modified inconsistently by BDZs: it is now believed that the presence of the $gamma_2$ subunit is strictly required for a clear BDZs subsensitivity to be expressed, although the type of alpha subunit may affect the affinity of the different ligands for the BDZ recognition site. Therefore, the coexpression of alpha, beta and $gamma_2$ subunits provides a BDZ modulatory site, the pharmacology of which is widely determined by the type of variants. The $alpha_1$ $beta_X$ $gamma_2$ receptor (where $beta_X$ is any beta subunit) thus possesses a pharmacological profile resembling the BDZ type I site displaying high affinity for triazolopiridazines, beta carbolines and imidazolopyridines. The other alpha variants with $beta_X$ and $gamma_2$ subunits constitute a receptor complex which exhibits pharmacological properties similar to the BDZ type II modulatory site. In other words, the combinations $alpha_2beta_Xgamma_2$, $alpha_3beta_Xgamma_2$ and $alpha_5beta_Xgamma_2$ all display the same ligand affinities of the BDZ II modulatory site.

However, heterogeneity within this group derives from the evidence that the imidazolopyridine, zolpidem differentiates among these sites, since it exhibits a reduced affinity at $alpha_2$ $alpha_3$)$beta_X gamma_2$ receptors (within the high nanomolar range) and almost no affinity to $alpha_5 beta_X gamma_2$ receptor sites (table 4). In this way, zolpidem recognizes three classes of modulatory sites:

- $alpha_1 beta_X gamma_2$ with high affinity
- $alpha_2$($alpha_3$)$beta_X gamma_2$ with intermediate affinity and
- $alpha_5 beta_X gamma_2$ with extremely low affinity.

Table 4 AFFINITY OF THREE OMEGA SITES AGONISTS FOR SIX SUBUNITS COMBINATIONS

	$alpha_1$ $beta_2$ $gamma_2$	$alpha_2$ $beta_2$ $gamma_2$	$alpha_3$ $beta_2$ $gamma_2$	$alpha_5$ $beta_2$ $gamma_2$	$alpha_4$ $beta_2$ $gamma_2$	$alpha_6$ $beta_2$ $gamma_2$
CL 218872	+++	+	+	++	-	-
2-Oxo-quazepam	++++	+++	+++	+++	-	-
Zolpidem	+++	++	++	-	n.d.	-

++++ very high affinity; +++ high affinity; ++ moderate affinity; + low affinity; — very low affinity; n.d., not determined.

At present, there is no known ligand which is able to differentiate between $alpha_2 beta_X gamma_2$ and $alpha_3 beta_X gamma_2$ modulatory sites.

Concerning the $alpha_4$ subunit, two isoforms, with different sequences, have been identified. One of these sequences seems to correspond to the $alpha_5$ subunit, while the pharmacology of the other remains to be investigated.

$GABA_A$ receptors containing the $alpha_6$ isoform ($alpha_6 beta_x gamma_2$), located only in the granular layer of the cerebellum, display a very low affinity for the classic BDZs or other ligands such as triazolopyridozines, imidazolopyridines and ciclopyrolones. The only compound to be recognized with high affinity by receptors containing $alpha_6$ is the partial inverse agonist sarmasenil (RO 154513), which can be used as a selective marker for the BDZ modulatory site with the $alpha_6$ subunit variant in the structure.

To summarize, four BDZ sites, now designed with novel nomenclature of omega modulatory sites, may be identified on the basis of structural characteristic and affinity properties.

The $omega_1$ modulatory site possesses affinity for all ligands including BDZs, beta-carbolines, cyclopyrrolones, imidazopyridines, imidazolopyrimidines, pyrazoloquinolinones, pyrazolopyridines and triazolopyridazines. It displays selectivity for beta-carbolines, triazolopyridazines (CL 218872) and imidazopyridines (zolpidem). It is likely that the omega$_1$ modulatory site possesses at least one alpha$_1$ subunit variant in its composition.

The omega$_2$ subtype is a modulatory site possessing alpha$_2$ and/or alpha$_3$ subtype variants, since recombinant GABA$_A$ receptors with alpha$_2$ or alpha$_3$ subunits cannot be differentiated pharmacologically. This site possesses affinity for all availablc ligands but, unlike the omega$_1$ site, does not display selectivity for any of them.

The omega$_5$ modulatory site is present in GABA$_A$ receptors that have the alpha$_5$ subunit variant in their structure. For the most part, it shows high affinity for synthetic ligands, with the exception of imidazolopyridines. This property distinguishes omega$_5$ pharmacologically from the alpha$_1$ and alpha$_2$ modulatory sites.

Omega$_6$ refers to the modulatory site bearing the alpha$_6$ variant subunit. It displays very low affinity for BDZs or other ligands such as triazolopyridazines, imidazopyridines and ciclopyrrolones, but can be recognized by imidazobenzodiazepinones, pyrazoloquinolinones and beta-carbolines. At this site, the imidazobenzopinone RO 15-4513 behaves as a selective marker, in the presence of diazepam (Turner et al., 1991).

The nomenclature and classification of BDZ modulatory sites are based on the pharmacological properties of the alpha subunit variants. Conversely, compared with the functions of the alpha isoforms, the precise roles of the beta, gamma and delta subunits are less well understood. Even though previous reports have indicated beta subunits as the site for GABA binding (Casalotti et al., 1986), recent evidence shows that channels composed exclusively of alpha or delta subunits can also be gated by GABA, indicating that the agonist binding site is not necessarily associated with beta subunits (Shivers et al., 1989; Ymer et al., 1989). Whether differences in the pharmacology of the receptor exist when variants of beta subunits are included in the alpha$_X$ beta$_X$ gamma$_2$ complex, require further investigation. Certainly, anomalous pharmacology is observed when gamma$_1$ replaces gamma$_2$ subunit. When the subunit composition alpha$_5$beta$_X$gamma$_1$ is expressed in cultured cells, the antagonist flumazenil and the inverse agonist DMCM (methyl 6,7 dimethoxy-4 ethyl beta carboline 3 carboxylate) both behave as agonists (Ymer et al., 1990). The modulation of Cl^- current by both BDZs and imidazopyridines is markedly reduced in GABA receptors carrying the gamma$_1$ subunit instead of the gamma$_2$ (Ymer et al., 1990). Thus, there is a tendency for alpidem and zolpidem to operate as negative modulators when applied to cells expressing alpha$_2$beta$_X$gamma$_1$ or alpha$_3$beta$_X$gamma$_1$ receptors (Puja et al., 1992). Finally, the function of the delta subunit in the receptor complex is still unclear compared to that of other subunit classes.

Brain Distribution of GABA Receptor Subunits

Regarding the brain location of the omega modulatory site subtypes, a large body of evidence suggests that each brain structure contains different molecular species of mRNA for GABA receptor subunits. Their relative abundance varies in different brain areas. The potency and efficacy of the regulation of $GABA_A$ receptor subtypes by various classes of BDZs depend on subunit assembly. Hence, the subtype of $GABA_A$ receptors that prevails in various brain areas influences the physiological and pharmacological nature of the GABAergic transmission in each region of the brain. In situ hybridization histochemistry has indicated that, at least in the brains of rats, $alpha_1$, $beta_2$ and $gamma_2$ are the most widely distributed isoforms, whereas other subunits display a more restricted and unique distribution (Shivers et al., 1989; Zhang et al., 1990; Olsen and Tobin, 1990).

Initial studies have suggested that mRNAs encoding the subunits exhibit heterogeneity in topographical distribution.

$Alpha_1$, $alpha_2$ and $alpha_4$ mRNAs are differently expressed along the neuraxis. Overall, $alpha_1$ mRNA is more abundant than $alpha_2$ or $alpha_4$ mRNAs. In many regions, all three mRNA species are co-expressed in the same structures, but often in different cell types and at different levels.

$Alpha_1$ mRNA is found in abundance, and is widely distributed with very high concentrations in the cerebellum and in all layers of the neocortex, medium concentrations in the mitral cells of the olfactory bulb and in the inferior culliculus, and in significant but lower concentrations in the globus pallidus, thalamus, some pyramidal cells of CA3 in the hippocampus, substantia nigra and some pontine nuclei. The caudate displays low levels, while there are no detectable levels at all in the spinal cord.

$Alpha_2$ mRNA is less abundant than $alpha_1$ mRNA and has a more limited distribution. The highest levels are in the olfactory bulb, hippocampal formation and the cranial motor nuclei. High to moderate labeling is found in several structures, including the anterior olfactory nuclei, olfactory tubercle, caudate-putamen, nucleus accumbens, piriform cortex and cerebral cortex.

$Alpha_4$ mRNA is less abundant than either $alpha_1$ and $alpha_2$ mRNA and is mainly expressed in neurons within the olfactory bulb and hippocampal formation. Moderate to low concentrations of $alpha_4$ mRNA are observed in the anterior olfactory nuclei, piriform cortex, cerebral cortex and amygdala.

$Alpha_5$ mRNA has a more restricted distribution, being detected in the olfactory bulb granular cells, deep cerebellar and brainstem nuclei. $Alpha_6$, the last of all the subunit isoforms studied to date, is the most restricted, and limited to the cerebellar granule cells.

The gamma type shows a distribution more typical of the pattern expected of the BDZ receptor from binding investigations, and parallels that of $alpha_1$ and $beta_2$ mRNAs. High concentrations of gamma type are seen in all layers of the neocortex, cerebellar Purkinje cells, mitral and tufted cell layers of the olfactory bulb and all hippocampal neurons. Medium concentrations are found in substantia nigra, globus pallidus and thalamus.

The delta mRNA is detected in areas showing high affinity muscimol binding without accompanying BDZ binding: lower binding in layer IV of the neocortex; a higher concentration in the internal granule layer of the olfactory bulb and cerebellum granule cell layer. Negligible concentrations are found in the olfactory bulb mitral cells, hippocampus pyramidal cells, cerebellum Purkinje cells, substantia nigra — typical $GABA_A$/omega sites regions (Richards et al., 1991). This suggests that the expression of $GABA_A$ receptor sub-units (and variants) in an area-specific manner determines the pharmacological profiles of GABA synapses in a given area.

It is now important to locate the BDZ modulatory sites within the human CNS.

Bibliography

Casalotti SD, Stephenson FA, Barnard EA: Separate subunits for agonist and benzodiazepine binding in gamma-aminobutyric $acid_A$ receptor oligomer. *Journal of Biological Chemistry* 261:15013-15016, 1986

Olsen RW and AJ Tobin: Molecular biology of $GABA_A$ receptors. Federation of *American Societies for Experimental Biology* 4:1469-1480, 1990

Puja G, Vicini S, Seeburg PN and Costa E: Influence of recombinant gamma aminobutyric $acid_A$ receptor subunit composition on the action of allosteric modulators of gamma-aminobutyric acid gated Cl^- currents. *Molecular Pharmacology* 39:691-696, 1992

Richards G, Schoch P and Haefely W "Benzodiazepine receptors: new vistas" seminars. In *The Neurosciences* 3:191-203, 1991

Schofield PR, Darlinson M, Fujita N, Burt D, Stephenson F, Rodriguez H, Rhee L, Ramachandran J, Reale V, Glencorse A, Seeburg PH and Barnarol EA: Sequence and functional expression of the $GABA_A$ receptor shows a ligand gated receptor super-family. *Nature* 32:221-227, 1987

Shivers BD, Killish I, Sprengel R, Sontheimer H, Mohler PR, Schofield PR and Seeburg PH: Two novel $GABA_A$ receptor subunits exist in distinct neuronal subpopulations. *Neuron* 3:327-337, 1989

Turner DM, Sapp DW and Olsen R: The benzodiazepine/alcohol antagonist RO 15-4513: binding to a GABA receptor subtype that is insensitive to diazepam. *Journal of Pharmacology and Experimental Therapeutics* 257:1236-1242, 1991

Ymer S, Draguhn A, Kohler M, Schoefield PR and Seeburg PH: Sequence and expression of a novel $GABA_A$ receptor subunit. *Federation of American Societies for Experimental Biology Lett* 258:119-122, 1989

Ymer S, Draghun A, Wisden W, Werner P, Keinanen K, Schofield PR, Sprengel R, Pritchett DB and Seeburg PH: Structural and functional characterization of the $gamma_1$ subunit of $GABA_A$/benzodiazepine receptors. *EMBO J* 9:3261-3267, 1990

Zhang JH, Sato M, Noguchi K and Tohyama M: The differential expression patterns of the mRNAs encoding beta subunits ($beta_1$, $beta_2$ and $beta_3$) of $GABA_A$ receptor in the olfactory bulb and its related areas in the rat brain. *Neuroscience Letters* 119:257-260, 1990

Group II
Compounds with Benzodiazepine-like Activity

This group includes compounds with a heterogeneous chemical structure, which share the characteristic of acting in vivo, similar to BDZs, by acting at the BDZ modulatory site in the brain.

Pharmacological tests in vivo and in vitro have made it possible to differentiate the action of these molecules and to make a distinction between agonists and antagonists, partial agonists and inverse agonists of BDZ receptors.

Agonists

Cyclopyrrolon

Among new anxiolytic drugs, cyclopyrrolones are of particular interest, because they have recently entered into wide clinical practice. Although chemically very different from BDZs, zopiclone and suriclone, the two most thoroughly studied compounds of the cyclopyrrolone family, possess the following properties (Julou et al., 1985):

1) the main type of activities characterizing the pharmacological profile of hypnotics or anxiolytics of the BDZ family
2) the capacity to displace BDZs from their sites
3) a therapeutic activity as an hypnotic (zopiclone) or anxiolytic (suriclone).

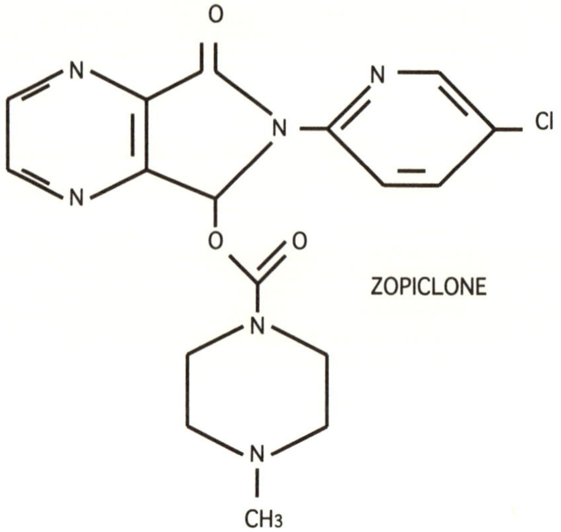

ZOPICLONE

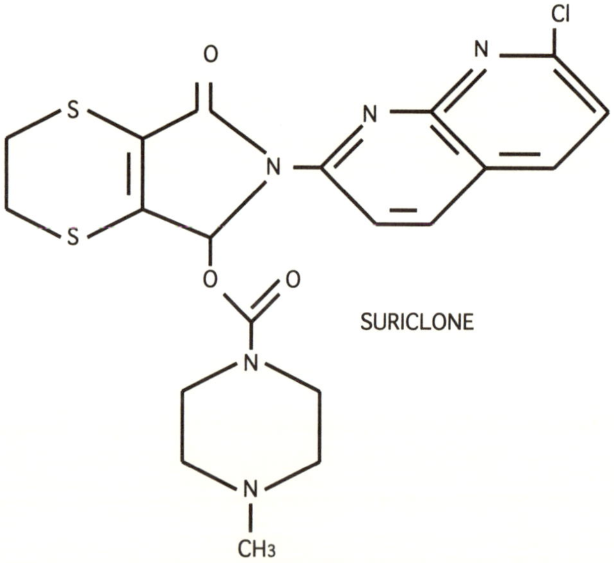

SURICLONE

Cyclopyrrolones are capable of displacing the BDZs from their binding site in the brain, suggesting the possibility that they might act at the same site. The regional distribution and pharmacologic specificity of cyclopyrrolone and BDZ binding sites are similar, giving rise to the hypothesis that cyclopyrrolone recognition sites reside on the BDZ receptor complex. Unlike classical BDZ agonists, the binding of cyclopyrrolone is not affected by GABA and pentobarbital. In addition, cyclopyrrolone binding sites are only weakly modulated by photoaffinity labeling with flunitrazepam. The association kinetics of cyclopyrrolones indicate that they provoke a conformational change upon binding to receptors. All findings suggest the assumption that cyclopyrrolones bind a site on the BDZ receptor complex linked allosterically to the recognition site for BDZs (Trifiletti and Snyder, 1984). Displacement studies indicate that unlike imidazopyridines but similar to BDZs, cyclopyrrolones do not discriminate among the central omega receptor site. Also, they do not possess peripheral binding sites (Doble et al., 1991).

Clinical tests have evidenced that zopiclone is active as an hypnotic in very low doses (7.5 mg), maintains its efficacy even in chronic administration, but does not enhance the effects of alcohol and or induce respiratory depression.

Suriclone has been shown to be an anxioselective agent in that it exhibits only weak sedative activity, and therefore it has been proposed as a suitable anxiolytic alternative to BDZs. At present, any judgement on its clinical efficacy has to await the results of large scale trials. Also, the interaction of suriclone with other CNS depressants is likely to be significantly less pronounced compared to the interactions of BDZs with these agents.

Suriclone appears to be an anxiolytic with limited effects on vigilance. Quantitative EEG investigations have shown that with doses of 0.5 mg and higher a typical anxiolytic EEG profile was obtained with a slower onset but a longer duration of effect than classical BDZs.

In generalized anxiety disorders, an anxiolytic effect is achieved with a dosage as low as 1 mg/die — with the best balance between effectiveness and tolerance yielded in a dose range of 1.2 to 1.8 mg/day. Suriclone is almost completely absorbed, and has a short distribution and elimination halflife. Like zopiclone, it is metabolized predominantly by three major pathways (oxidation, demethylation and decarboxylation). Neither the drug nor its derivatives are detectable in plasma 48 hours after administration. Initial findings on dependence potential have shown that suriclone does not induce BDZ-like physical dependence in either humans and experimental animals (Piot et al., 1990). This would give cyclopyrrolones a significant advantage over BDZs and would suggest these drugs have a potential therapeutic usefulness against anxiety (Oli et al., 1992; Kelly et al., 1990).

Following a single oral dose of 7.5 mg, zopiclone is readily absorbed with peak-plasma concentrations of 60-70 μg/l reached within 0.5-1.5 hours. More than 93% of absorption is complete one hour after administration. The bioavailability of an oral dose is approximately 85%, suggesting no significant "first-pass" effect. Total bioavailability appears to be independent of dosage, and a linear correlation exists between plasma levels and dose in a wide range. The drug exhibits a first order kinetics, as the drug, following i.v. administration, penetrates tissues including the brain, very rapidly. The distribution volume estimated after i.v. or increasing oral doses is about 100 l. Zopiclone is excreted in the breast-milk with a milk/plasma ratio averaging 0.5. The curve showing milk drug concentrations over time parallels that seen in the plasma. The elimination half-life of zopiclone and its active N-oxide metabolite ranges from 3.4 to 6.1 hours. After i.v. administration the drug undergoes biphasic elimination with a mean half-life of about 5 hours. Sex and multiple dose schedule do not significantly affect zopiclone kinetics. The short elimination half-life is prolonged in patients with severe liver diseases and in elderly subjects to about 8 hours, but is not slower in patients with moderate renal failure. Zopiclone undergoes extensive metabolism in the liver — only 4 to 5% of the dose is excreted unchanged in the urine. The oxidation of the side chain generates the less active N-oxide derivative, which accounts for 10% of the dose. The elimination half-life of this metabolite is similar to the parent drug. A second route involves demethylation to inactive N-desmethyl zopiclone, which accounts for 15% of a dose. Both derivatives are excreted in the urine. Ester hydrolysis involving oxidative decarboxylation of 50% of a dose generates inactive metabolites partly eliminated via the lung as carbon dioxide.

Plasma clearance of zopiclone is about 14 l/hour in healthy volunteers and is not increased by dialysis. What is interesting is that coadministration of alcohol, H_2 antagonist, tricyclic antidepressant do not seem to affect zopiclone pharmacokinetics. Conversely, metoclopramide, atropine and all drugs which influence gastric motility may alter zopiclone plasma concentrations.

Bibliography

Doble A, Canton T, Piot O, Zundel JL, Stutzmann JM, Cotrel C and Blanchard JC: The pharmacology of cyclopyrrolone derivatives acting at the $GABA_A$/benzodiazepine receptor". *7th Sardinian conference of neuroscience —GABAergic synaptic transmission: molecular, pharmacological and clinical aspects, Cagliari* 62AB:344P.62, 1991

Julou L, Blanchard JC and Breyfus JF: Pharmacological and clinical studies of cyclopyrrolones: zopiclone and suriclone. *Pharmacology Biochemistry and Behavior* 23:653-659, 1985

Kelly F, O'Grady J and Champey Y: Zopiclone. *Lancet* 335:1033-1034, 1990

Oli JP, Truffinet P, Guillet P and Pilate C: The anxiolytic efficacy of suriclone. *Clinical Neuropharmacology* 15:170B, 1992

Piot O, Betschart J, Stutzmann JM and Blanchard JC: Cyclopyrrolones, unlike some benzodiazepines, do not induce physical dependence in mice. *Neuroscience Letters* 117:140-143, 1990

Trifiletti RR and Snyder SH: Anxiolytic cyclopyrrolones zopiclone and suriclone bind to a novel site linked allosterically to benzodiazepines. *Molecular Pharmacology* 26:458-469, 1984

Imidazopyridine

Alpidem and zolpidem are the most interesting among these emerging compounds. They act through BDZ receptor subtypes, which according to Langer and Arbilla (1988), have been named as omega receptors. Alpidem appears to have a more pronounced anxiolytic activity, while zolpidem has mainly hypnotic properties.

Zolpidem

Zolpidem is an imidazopyridine, a chemically novel nonbenzodiazepine hypnotic agent. It interacts at the benzodiazepine omega$_1$ subtype in the brain — its regional location of zolpidem binding paralleling that of the omega$_1$ subtype, predominant in cortex, cerebellum, substantia nigra and pallidum. Compatible with these sites of action, zolpidem exhibits a pharmacological profile different from BDZs. Indeed, it possesses sedative activity which predominates over the anti-convulsivant and anxiolytic effects.

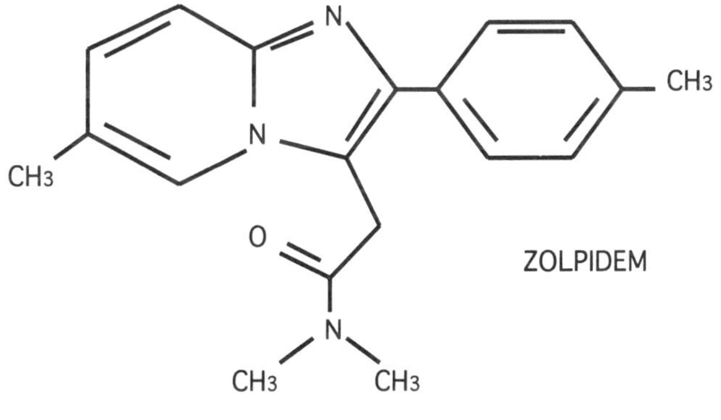

ZOLPIDEM

Zolpidem is devoid of any myorelaxant property. The lack of myorelaxant effects is related to its weak affinity for the co-subtype (omega$_2$) localized in the spinal cord responsible for the muscle tone, whereas the sedative action is linked to its high intrinsic activity at, and selective affinity for, the omega$_1$ receptor site (Langer and Arbilla, 1988; Depoortere et al., 1986).

Zolpidem is readily absorbed from the gastrointestinal tract, even if a substantial pre-systemic biodegradation results in an absolute bioavailability of approximately 70% following oral doses of 5 to 20 mg. Peak plasma concentrations of about 200 μg/l are obtained within 2.2 hours following a single oral dose of 20 mg. Absorption is not significantly altered during prolonged administration, as peak serum levels of 200 μg/l are yielded within 2.3 hours on day 15 of the treatment. Zolpidem is highly bound the plasma proteins with a free fraction ranging around 8%. Although it is extensively linked to serum albumin, zolpidem concentrates initially in glandular tissue, and in fact with the lowest concentration in the brain it is readily eliminated with only negligible amounts detected in non secretory tissue 3 hours following the administration.

Brain/plasma concentration ratios in animals average 0.4, with unchanged zolpidem accounting for between 50 and 80% of the amount found in CNS. The drug is secreted in small amounts in breast milk when administered to a lactating woman.

Three major metabolites of zolpidem have been identified in man. None displays pharmacological activity. The major degradative pathways involve oxidation of the methyl group of the phenyl or imidazopyridine group, to generate carboxylic acids, and hydroxylation of the imidazolopyridine nucleus. A minor route includes oxidation of the methyl groups on the substituted amide. Unchanged drug is detected in very negligible amounts (<1%).

The elimination half-life of zolpidem ranges from 1.4 to 2.5 hours in healthy subjects; estimated systemic clearance is 0.25 l/h/Kg. The distribution volume is calculated around 0.55 l/Kg following an 8 mg i.v. injection of zolpidem. Serious liver diseases and renal failure result in a prolonged elimination half-life, and therefore dosage reductions are required. Zolpidem is not removed by dialysis. Age appears to affect zolpidem elimination, since a longer half-life has been reported in the elderly compared to children. Sex may also influence zolpidem pharmacokinetics, as higher plasma concentration may occur in women. Thus, age and gender may influence the incidence of unwanted effects, whereas food and coadministration of a number of drugs (including H_2-antagonists, warfarin, haloperidol and imipramine) do not affect zolpidem pharmacokinetics.

Alpidem

Alpidem is an imydazopyridine, a chemically non-BDZ compound which displays a selective affinity for omega$_1$ receptor sites, and preferentially binds to the brain areas enriched with this receptor subtype such as sensory-motor cortex and cerebellum (Langer and Arbilla, 1988).

Although the intrinsic mechanism of action resembles that of BDZs, its differential regional selectivity may account for its original pharmacological profile. In addition to its anticonvulsant property, alpidem has been reported to possess anxiolytic effects, as shown in several different animal models. However, unlike BDZs which exhibit central depressant effects at doses within the anxiolytic range, alpidem is virtually devoid of sedative and myorelaxant activity, and does not produce any memory and learning impairment at doses displaying anti-anxiety effects. The lack of myorelaxant and amnesic activity is related to the low affinity of alpidem for the co-receptor subtypes located into the spinal cord and the hippocampus. In contrast to its failure to affect muscle tone and cognitive function, the fact that alpidem does not exert central depressant activity is not related to the selectivity of binding for omega$_1$ receptor subtype, since other imidazopyridines with a similar receptor affinity possess strong sedative activity — unlike alpidem. The discrepancy in sedative potential among imidazopyridines may be explained by the difference in their intrinsic activity: as a result, because alpidem possesses a weak intrinsic activity it behaves as a partial agonist and induces negligible sedation (Zivkovic et al., 1991; Zivkovic et al., 1992).

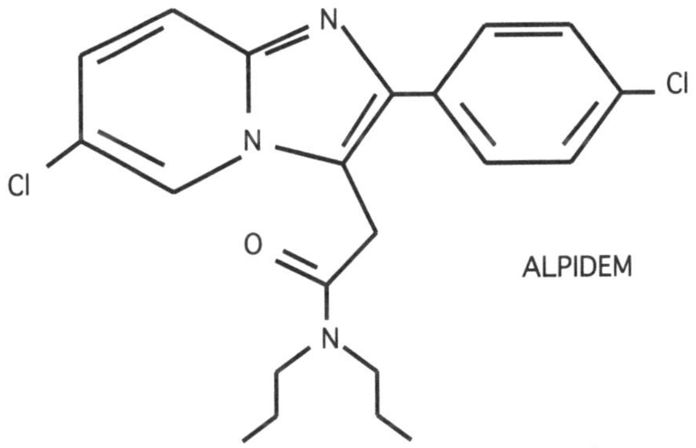

ALPIDEM

Another difference between alpidem and BDZs concerns the propensity to develop tolerance and physical dependence on long-term usage. The receptor selectivity coupled with a weak intrinsic activity may account for the low potential of alpidem to induce tolerance and dependence upon prolonged administration. Alpidem is characterized by linear non-saturable kinetics in humans.

Peak plasma concentrations are reached within 1.4-2 hours following oral intake, with a bioavailability of 30-36%. Alpidem is highly bound to plasma proteins and has a terminal half-life of 15-24 hours in normal volunteers. Pharmacokinetic investigations show that it represents a minor component in the plasma which is widely metabolized. Three main processes of biotransformation have been defined and beta-derivatives identified:

a) aliphatic oxidation of the substituted amide side chains

b) aromatic oxidation of the imidazopyridine mojety
c) N-dealkylation

Whether any of the metabolically generated products possess pharmacological activity is now under investigation.

The urinary elimination of alpidem is very low in humans and in laboratory animals, whereas most of the oral dose is excreted in faeces.

Doses suggested for adults range between 25-150 mg/day (Mush et al., 1988). This drug recently has been withdrawn from the market for its toxicity.

Triazolopyridazines

CL 218872 shows some structural similarity with purines, and is very active as an anxiolytic in the conflict test and as an antagonist of pentilentetrazol-induced seizures. It is considered a selective antianxiety agent because it does not produce sedation and ataxia (Zivkovic et al., 1992). The high hepatic toxicity in animals has however, prevented further pharmacological tests in man.

Bibliography

Depoortere H, Zivkovic B, Lloyd KG, Sanger DJ, Perrault G, Langer SZ and Bartholini G: Zolpidem, a novel non-benzodiazepine hypnotic 1. Neuropharmacological and behavioral effects. *Journal of Pharmacology and Experimental Therapeutics* 237:649-658, 1986

Langer SE and Arbilla S: Imidazopyridines as a tool for the characterization of benzodiazepine receptors: A proposal for a pharmacological classification as omega receptor subtypes. *Pharmacology Biochemistry and Behavior* 29:763-766, 1988

Musch B, Morselli PL and Priore P: Clinical studies with the new anxiolytic alpidem in anxious patients: an overview of the European Experiences. *Pharmacology Biochemistry and Behavior* 29:803-806, 1988

Zivkovic B, Perrault G and Sanger DJ: Pharmacological and behavioural profile of alpidem as an anxiolytic. In: *Biological Psychiatry*. Racagni G et al. (eds.) Elsevier Science Publishers B.V, vol. 1, pp. 686-688, 1991

Zivkovic B, Perrault G and Sanger DJ: Receptor subtype-selective drugs: a new generation of anxiolytics and hypnotics. In: *Target receptor for anxiolytics and hypnotics: from molecular pharmacology to therapeutics*. Mendlewicz J and Racagni G (eds.) Karger, Basel, pp. 55-73, 1992

Partial Agonists

Up until the last decade, it was commonly believed that the structure of BDZs was a condition strictly required for the recognition of and the binding to the BDZ receptor site. However, molecules chemically unrelated with BDZs have since been proved to display a pharmacological profile similar to BDZs via the interaction at the same receptor site. It has been suggested therefore that the term "BDZ receptor ligands" should refer to all molecules that, irrespective of their structural characteristics, modulate GABA transmission by interacting at a BDZ recognition site.

As already described, the cyclopyrrolone zopiclone was the first compound to be identified that while not structurally a BDZ did show the typical BDZ-like profile of activity and affinity for the BDZ receptor. Since 1980, and the advent of ligands from the class of beta-carbolines, several other chemical classes have been found to contain derivatives with affinity to the BDZ receptor site, viz. triazolopyridazines, pyrazoloquinolines and imidazopyridines. These compounds share positive and negative properties with classic BDZs.

"BDZ receptor ligands" produce a variety of pharmacological effects, and a number of in vitro and in vivo biochemical techniques and behavioral paradigms in animals have been devised to quantify their antianxiety, anticonvulsant, sedative and myorelaxant properties.

The in vivo binding techniques combined with either the electrophysiological chloride influx measurements or appropriate behavioral testing allow us to determine the receptor occupancy required to yield a given response with the compound under investigation. It has been demonstrated that a drug acting as a full agonist at BDZ receptor inhibits pentylenetetrazole-induced convulsion when the receptor occupancy is about 25%, whereas anti-anxiety activity is not yielded until 60% of the receptor population is occupied. Ataxia occurs at still higher occupancy.

Clearly the ability to estimate the receptor occupancy required for a given effect allows the comparison of different ligands and the definition of compounds with high and low efficacy. Low efficacy compounds or partial agonists induce smaller responses in their target cells than full agonists at the same fractional receptor occupancy. Partial agonists would therefore be expected to have a pharmacological profile restricted to those effects normally seen with a full agonist, and would not be able to provide the receptor stimulation required to produce the ataxic effects. This is of particular clinical interest since partial agonists in anxiolytic and anticonvulsant doses produce less sedation (with less impairment of learning and memory) muscle relaxation (and ataxia), tolerance and physical dependence.

Bretazenil

Bretazenil is an imidazo-benzodiazepine compound displaying features characteristic of a BDZ receptor partial agonist. Its pharmacological profile is best shown by fractional receptor occupancy in relation to fractional effect curves in a variety of test situations compared with full agonists. Facilitation of GABA-induced chloride conductance is less marked with bretazenil than with full agonists. In fact, full agonists result in half maximal-facilitation at about 25% receptor occupancy, whereas bretazenil requires over 90% occupancy to yield about 25% of the maximal effect of a full agonist.

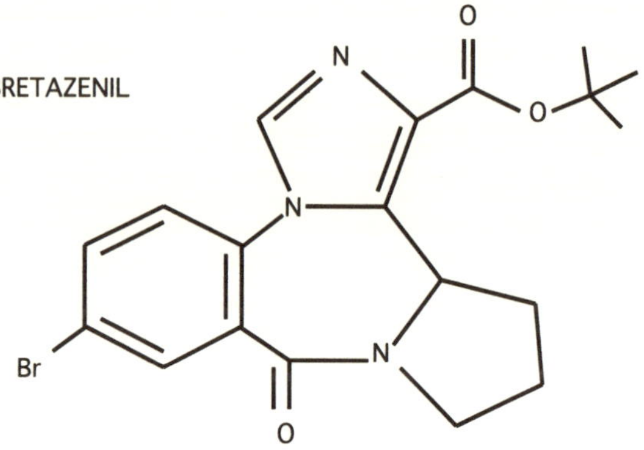

Studies using in vivo labelling of cerebral BDZ receptor (positron emission tomography studies) have shown that bretazenil requires higher fractional receptor occupancy and various pharmacological effects in experimental animals reveals a low occupancy by a full agonist for anxiolytic and anticonvulsant effects, and somewhat higher occupancy for moderate and severe sedation. Bretazenil requires a higher fractional receptor occupancy than a full agonist for equivalent anxiolytic and anticonvulsant effects. Severe sedation and motor impairment are not obtained with this compound even at receptor saturating doses (Haefely et al., 1990).

In clinical trials, bretazenil shows the typical separation between various effects and, in the presence of a full agonist even antagonises its sedative and ataxic effects (Martin et al., 1988). In clinical practice, the starting dose of bretazenil is 0.5 mg, which can be gradually increased up to 4 mg/day, even if the common daily dose is 1.5 mg.

Abecarnil

Abecarnil, a new beta-carboline derivative with high affinity for BDZ receptors, possesses anxiolytic and anticonvulsant properties, but with considerably reduced myorelaxant effects compared to diazepam.

Like bretazenil, abecarnil appears to be from 2 to 10 times more potent than diazepam in most rodent tests of anxiolytic activity and in reducing locomotor activity in animals thoroughly habituated to the test chamber. In tests for motor coordination, abecarnil, in contrast to full agonist diazepam, displays only negligible activity. The enhancement of abecarnil binding by GABA (GABA shift) is less marked than the effect of GABA on diazepam binding. Fractional receptor occupancy at comparable end-points of pharmacological activity is much higher with abecarnil than with full agonists. This profile of pharmacological activity suggests that abecarnil behaves as a partial agonist at central BDZ receptors (Stephen et al., 1990) and predicts that it may be a clinically useful anti-anxiety agent with a reduced incidence of undesirable effects compared to conventional BDZ derivatives.

In the cases of bretazenil and abecarnil, the separation of wanted and unwanted effects has been explained in terms of partial agonism. However, the existence of BDZ receptor subtypes could provide a further explanation. Indeed, identification of several variants of the $GABA_A$ receptor sub-units may offer the possibility of different BDZ receptor ligands in terms both of affinity and extent or direction of activation. Therefore, the selective ligand affinity to particular receptor subtypes does not necessarily represent an alternative to partial agonism, but it does complicate the situation by suggesting that both the affinity and intrinsic efficacy of any ligand for any receptor variant have to be taken into account in order to evaluate the pharmacological profile of anxiolytic compounds.

Bibliography

Haefely W, Martin JR and Schoch P: Novel anxiolytics that act as partial agonists at benzodiazepine receptors. *Trends in Pharmacological Sciences* 11:452-456, 1990

Martin JR, Pieri L, Bonetti EP, Schaffner R, Burkard WP, Cumin R and Haefely W: RO 16-6028: a novel anxiolytic agent acting as a partial agonist at the benzodiazepine receptor. *Pharmacopsychiatry* 21:360-362, 1988

Stephen DN, Schneider HH, Kehr W, Jansen LH, Petersen E and Honore J: Abecarnil, a metabolically stable, anxioselective beta-carboline acting at benzodiazepine receptor. *Journal of Pharmacology and Experimental Therapeutics* 253:334-343, 1990

Benzodiazepine Receptor Antagonists

During recent years, there has been an increase in knowledge of the relationship between the structure of BDZ receptor ligands and their pharmacological properties. This has led to the development of a wide spectrum of compounds which interact at BDZ receptors with different intrinsic efficacy. The intrinsic property of BDZ ligands, which determines the direction and intensity of allosteric modulation, is called intrinsic efficacy according to basic pharmacology.

BDZ receptor ligands exhibit a continuum of intrinsic efficacies: from full positive intrinsic efficacy on the extreme left (resulting in anxiolytic, anticonvulsant, sedative and myorelaxant effects) to full negative intrinsic efficacy on the extreme right (anxiogenic, convulsant, stimulant and spasmogenic effect). In the center, are pure antagonists with zero intrinsic efficacy. Thus, the BDZ receptor also recognizes ligand without modulatory activity which however, competitively blocks the effects of agonist and inverse agonist (Haefely, 1990).

Flumazenil belongs to this latter group; with approximately the equivalent potency as an antagonist as diazepam as an agonist (Amrein et al., 1987).

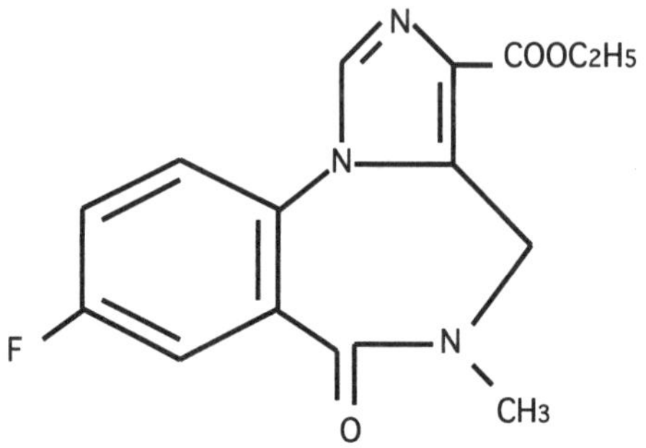

N N $COOC_2H_5$ F O N CH_3

FLUMAZENIL

In a variety of tests in rodents, flumazenil, a 1,4 imidazobenzodiazepine derivative, 0.3-30 mg/Kg i.v. or 2.5 mg intracerebroventricularly has been reported to antagonize both the central effects of BDZ agonists (such as diazepam, midazolam, lorazepam) and inverse agonists (such as dimethoxy-ethyl-carbomethoxy-beta-carboline: DMCM). The antagonist effect of flumazenil is specific for central BDZ receptor sites (File and Pellow, 1986). In fact, in binding investigations in both humans and rodents, it inhibits the pharmacological effect (including cognitive impairment, motor function sedation) when co-administered or administered at various intervals. The duration and intensity of flumazenil antagonism of agonists and inverse agonists central effects appear, in some instances, to be dose-dependent. The efficacy of flumazenil in reversing the effect of BDZs during recovery has been reported in patients using BDZs for diagnostic procedures or for anaesthesia.

Its utility in the initial management of BDZ overdose has been repeatedly confirmed, whereas its efficacy in alleviating hepatic encephalopathy is still controversial (Klotz and Walker, 1989; Skolnick, 1989). Flumazenil is clearly very useful in treating drug poisoning when BDZs are the major component (Aarseth et al., 1988).

By virtue of its pharmacological profile, flumazenil represents a useful and well tolerated tool in all clinical situation requiring rapid reversal of BDZ central unwanted actions.

The dose of flumazenil should be tailored individually to achieve the desired effects. Commonly, doses of 0.3-0.6 mg i.v. are enough to reduce sedation in patients sedated with BDZs, while 0.5-1 mg is the appropriate dose to completely reverse the effect of a therapeutic dose of a BDZ agonist.

In patients unconscious from a drug overdose, the failure of 5 mg of flumazenil to improve the level of consciousness suggests the involvement of toxics other than BDZs. The flumazenil is transient (not exceeding 1 hour), so repeated low doses are required (Klotz et al., 1984). Administering flumazenil to these subjects does not eliminate the need for adequate laboratory and clinical monitoring.

Clinically, flumazenil is administered by i.v. route.

Steady-state plasma concentrations are achieved in 1.5 hours. in normal volunteers, who receive a loading dose of 1-3 mg followed by the same dose in one hour and are about 13-39 μg/l.

The protein binding of flumazenil in plasma is 40-50%.

Its maximum distribution in the brain is achieved 5-8 minutes after i.v. administration. Flumazenil is degraded to the inactive free carboxylic acid and the corresponding glucuronide. Total body clearance is moderately high at about 55-65 l/h and elimination half-life is short (0.7-1.2 hours). This may explain why repeated injections or i.v. infusion are appropriate (Klotz and Kanto, 1988).

Bibliography

Aarseth HP, Bredesen JE, Grynne B, Lyngdal PT, Storstein L, et al.: Benzodiazepine-receptor antagonist, a clinical double blind study. *Clinical Toxicology* 26:283-292, 1988

Amrein R, Leishman B, Benzinger C and Roncari G: Flumazenil in benzodiazepine antagonism: actions and clinical use in intoxications and anaesthesiology. *Medical Toxicology* 2:411-429, 1987

File SE and Pellow S: Intrinsic actions of the benzodiazepine receptor antagonist Ro 15-1788. *Psychopharmacology* 88:1-11, 1986

Haefely WE: The $GABA_A$-benzodiazepine receptor complex and anxiety. In: Sartorius N et al. (eds.) *Anxiety: psychobiological and clinical perspectives*. HPC Chap. 3 pp. 23-36, 1990

Klotz U and Kanto J: Pharmacokinetics and clinical use of flumazenil (Ro 15-1788). *Clinical Pharmacokinetics* 14:1-2, 1988

Klotz U and Walker S: Flumazenil and hepatic encephalopathy. *Lancet* 1:155-156, 1989

Klotz U, Zielger G and Reimann IW: Pharmacokinetics of the selective benzodiazepine antagonist Ro 15-1788 in man. *European Journal of Clinical Pharmacology* 27:115-117, 1984

Skolnick P: The gamma-aminobutyric acid ($GABA_A$)-benzodiazepine receptor complex" In Jones EA, moderator. The gamma-aminobutyric acid A ($GABA_A$) receptor complex and hepatic encephalopathy: some recent advances. *Annals of Internal Medicine* 110:532-546, 1989

Group III
Compounds Acting on Non-Benzodiazepine Receptors

Serotonin and Anxiety

The psychobiological basis of mental illness is currently investigated by extrapolating neurochemical data from the mechanism of action of psychotropic agents. This approach has been used for anxiety disorders, and thus anxiolytic drugs can be considered as tools for understanding the biology of anxiety. The validity of this approach rests on the pharmacological specificity of the drugs used in the treatment of anxiety, and on the correlation between the neurochemical changes induced by the drug and its ability to control the sintomatology. However, the pharmacological profile of the most commonly prescribed anxiolytic agents, the BDZs, is extremely wide, since they possess — in addition to the anxiolytic effect — myorelaxant, sedative, hypnotic and anticonvulsant properties. Therefore, it may be difficult to separate the anxiolytic effect from the other effects displayed by these drugs, even though promising results have been achieved in this direction. A large body of evidence suggests that the mechanism of action of BDZs is related to their ability to bind a specific modulatory site on the GABA receptor complex, resulting in increased Cl^- inward flow and subsequent potentiation of the GABA function. Nevertheless, the concept that only one neurotransmitter system is involved in an important way in the pathophysiology of anxiety and in its relief has to be revised — mainly in the light of the recent discovery of anxiolytic agents, such as buspirone, gepirone, and ipsapirone which do not interact at omega modulatory sites. Since these anxiolytic drugs behave as serotoninergic partial agonists, abnormalities in serotoninergic neurotransmission have been suggested in the neurochemical alterations of anxiety disorders. Original investigations have supported the view that serotoninergic neurotransmission plays an important role in the pathophysiology of anxiety. Behaviourally, conflict tests in laboratory animals have been utilized as tools to quantify anxiolytic effects.

Changes in central serotoninergic transmission result in clear cut effects on the behavioural model of anxiety. Depletion of the brain serotonin (5-HT) content induced by the synthesis inhibitor parachlorophenilalanine can mimic the anxiolytic drug effects (Wise et al., 1972). Moreover, a strong anxiolytic effect is provoked by the selective 5-HT neurotoxin 5,6-dihydroxytryptamine (Iversen, 1984). In similar animal investigations, the injection of 5-HT intraventricular can antagonize the anticonflict effect of BDZs (Wise et al., 1972). It has been known for some time that BDZs also reduce 5-HT turnover in the brain (Stein et al., 1975). Metabolic studies have demonstrated that BDZs markedly reduce 5-HT content in the CNS (Saner and Pletscher, 1979). A number of GABA agonists have been reported to antagonize the accumulation of 5-hydroxytryptophan, a precursor in the synthesis process of 5-HT in serotonergic neurons (Nishikawa and Scatton, 1985). A large body of literature has emerged suggesting the involvement of 5-HT in anxiety and the modifications of 5-HT mechanisms to be an approach to the development of novel anxiolytic agents.

Interest has been expanded by the reported clinical anxiolytic effects of buspirone that, in addition to many pharmacological properties, interact with 5-HT_{1A} receptors (Glaser and Traber, 1983). There is some evidence from animal tests (Colpaert, 1985) and clinical trials that the 5-HT_2 antagonist ritanserin also possesses anxiolytic properties, if only over a narrow dose range. Finally, the 5-HT_3 antagonist GR 380327 has been reported to display anxiolytic effects in some animal models (Jones et al., 1988). It seems therefore that a variety of compounds, which behave as agonists or antagonists at central 5-HT receptor sites, show anxiolytic properties. The development of such agents is related to an explosive interest in, and extensive literature on the characterization of up to seven 5-HT receptor subtypes. Currently, the "recepterology" of 5-HT identifies the following receptors: 5-HT_{1A}; 5-HT_{1B}; 5-HT_{1C}; 5-HT_{1D}; 5-HT_2; 5-HT_3 and 5-HT_4. In addition, many others have been proposed (e.g. 5-HT_{1E}; 5-HT_{1P}; 5-HT_{1R}; 5-HT_{3A}; 5-HT_{3B}; 5HT_{3C}) but further investigations are required before they can be definitely identified (table 1).

Table 1 CLASSIFICATION, LOCALIZATION AND FUNCTION OF 5-HT RECEPTORS

Receptor type	Localization	Function
5-HT_1		
5-HT_{1A}	Mainly in the CNS, somatodendritic autoreceptor, postsynaptic in 5-HT terminal regions	Neuronal hyperpolarization, inhibition 5-HT neuronal firing, induction of specific behaviours, neuroendocrine response in man, adaptive-protective response to adversive stimulation
5-HT_{1B}	Only found in rodents, terminal autoreceptor	Inhibition of neurotransmitter (5-HT) release
5-HT_{1C}	Brain regions and choroid plexus	Augmentation of PI turnover, Induction of specific behaviour, feeding, anxiety
5-HT_{1D}	CNS, terminal autoreceptor (man), heteroreceptors on nigral terminals, postsynaptic in the striatum	Inhibition of neurotransmitter (5-HT) release
5-HT_1-like	Intracranial vasculature	Contraction
5-HT_1-like	Vascular smooth muscle, gastrointestinal smooth muscle	Relaxation
5-HT_2	CNS, postsynaptic in hippocampus, frontal cortex, spinal cord. Vascular smooth muscle, platelets lung, gastrointestinal tract	Induction of specific behaviour, slow wave sleep in man, vasoconstriction, platelet aggregation, bronchoconstriction
5-HT_3	Peripheral and central neurons, area postrema, limbic regions, nucleus tractus solitarius	Depolarization, activation of sensory afferents, control of emesis, modulation of neuro-transmitter release (dopamine, acetylcho line in limbic areas)

Table 1 CLASSIFICATION, LOCALIZATION AND FUNCTION OF 5-HT RECEPTORS ***(continued)***

Receptor type	Localization	Function
5-HT_4	CNS, hippocampus (guinea pig), colliculus (mouse), gastrointestinal tract, heart	Augmentation of cAMP, activation of neurotransmitter release

Figure 1 shows a serotoninergic synapse with A) the main steps of 5-HT metabolism and B) a putative localization of receptor subtypes and related intracellular mechanisms of signal transduction.

In order to study the mechanisms by which the various 5-HT receptor subtypes can mediate anxiety, site-selective agents are needed. The ideal situation would be the availability of high specific compounds for each receptor subtype. Unfortunately, this is not the case, since many agents proposed as selective have been demonstrated to possess only a rather marginal specificity. This complicates the interpretation of the experimental results and adds complexity to the understanding of the role of the various receptor subtypes in the pathophysiology of anxiety.

Studies of 5-HT_{1A} receptor agonists, partial agonists and antagonists in anxiety tests have given conflicting results. For example, 8-OH-DPAT has shown anxiolytic, anxiogenic, and no activity, depending on the test and the authors (Engel, 1986; Critchley and Handley, 1987; Carli et al., 1988; Pellow et al., 1987; Critchley and Handley, 1989).

The 5-HT_{1A} full agonist, 5 methoxy-N,N-dimethyltryptamine (5-MeO-DMT), LY 165163 (1-(mtrifluoromethylphenyl)-4-p aminophenylethyl) piperazine and (-) and (+) MDL72832 have been reported to be anxiogenic in various animal models (Critchley and Handley,1986; Critchley and Handley,1987).

Buspirone reduces aggression and produces anti-conflict activity both in rodents and primates (Merlo-Pinch and Samanin, 1986). Buspirone and diazepam exhibit a similar degree of anticonflict potency in the Vogel test, which is able to identify potential antianxiety substances (Barrett,1991).

In contrast, buspirone appears to be inactive in several models of anxiety where diazepam is active. For instance, buspirone does not work in the punished drinking test in the rat (Budhram et al., 1986) and it is inactive in the punished lever pressing test (Howard and Pollard, 1990). Its direct infusion into median raphe produced increases in exploratory behaviour in rodents

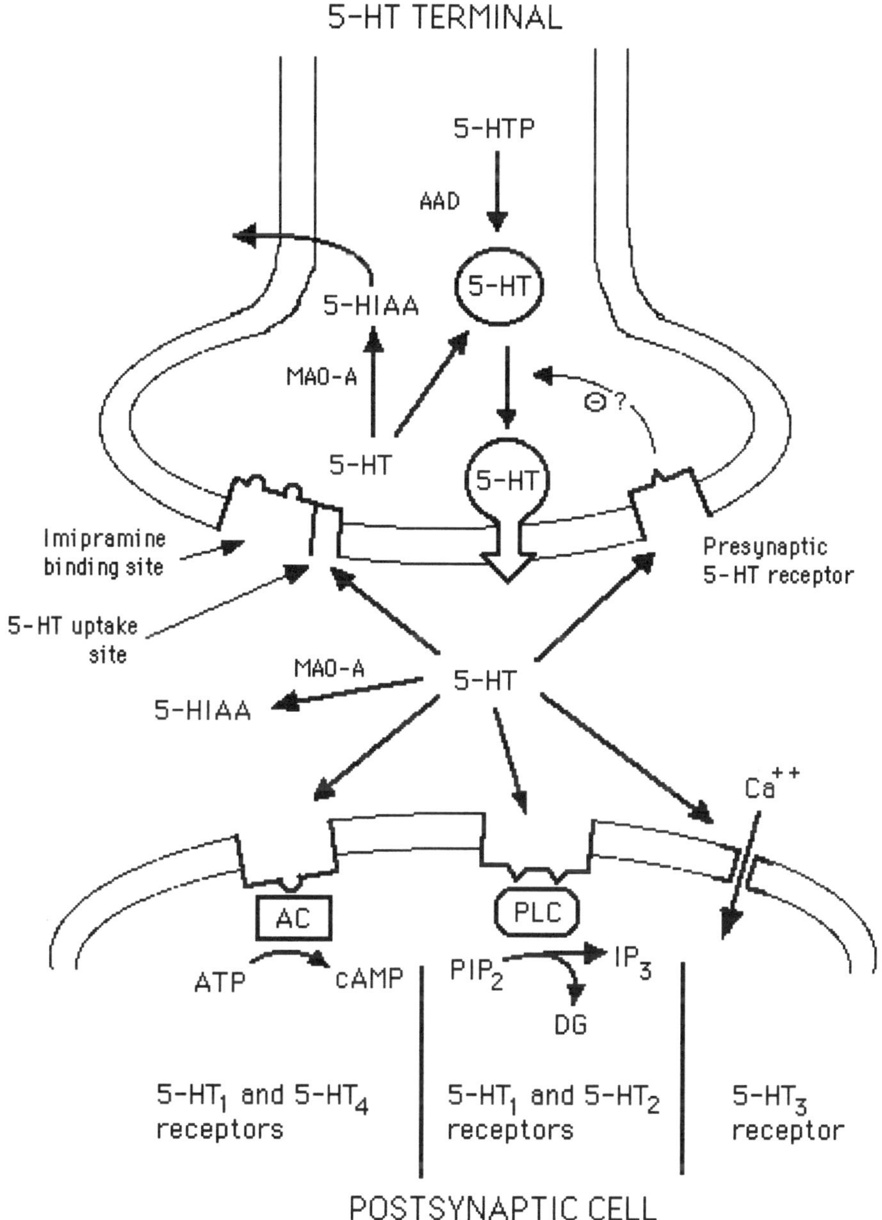

Fig. 1 Schematic representation of a serotoninergic synapse. AAD, aromatic aminoacid decarboxylase; AC, adenylate cyclase; ATP, adenosine triphosphate; cAMP, cyclic adenosine monophosphate; DG, diacylglycerol; 5-HIAA, 5-hydroxyindoleacetic acid; 5-HTP, 5-hydroxytryptophan; IP_3, inositol-1,4,5-triphosphate; MAO-A, monoamine oxidase A; PIP_2, phosphatidylinositol-4,5-bisphosphate ; PLC, phospholipase C.

with integrity of serotoninergic pathways, whereas 5,7-dihydroxytryptamine treatment reduced the anticonflict effect of buspirone (Eison et al., 1986).

Other 5-HT_{1A} partial agonists, such as ipsapirone, gepirone and MDL730051 have been reported to display anxiolytic properties in a number of animal models, including conflict test (Moser et al., 1988), social interaction test (Higgins, 1987) and elevated plus maze test (Critchly and Handley, 1989). However, other paradigms failed to establish a clear anxiolytic activity (Briley and Chopin, 1991).

While some studies have difficulties in confirming that 5-HT_{1A} partial agonists are active in certain behavioural tests predictors of anxiolytic properties, there is enough evidence to suggest that buspirone possesses antianxiety activity in humans. On this basis, the hypothesis that animal conflict tests may investigate impulsive behaviour rather than anxiety has to be taken into account (Treit, 1985).

Even though buspirone is apparently as effective as diazepam at controlling anxiety in humans, its pharmacological profile is far different from BDZs.

Compared to BDZs, buspirone shows a delayed onset of action (15 days or more) and is more effective in subjects who have never been treated previously with anxiolytic drugs (Goa and Ward, 1986). Interestingly, buspirone has not yet been found to induce tolerance or to potentiate ethanol. Similar results were found in clinical trials involving the use of gepirone and ipsapirone (more selective agents devoid of any dopaminergic activity) (Traber and Glaser, 1987). The efficacy of these compounds is reported to be independent from any history of previous anxiolytic medication. A large body of clinical evidence therefore indicates that the partial 5-HT_{1A} agonists appear to be as potent as classical 1,4-BDZs in the relief of anxiety, with minimal effects on levels of alertness, coordination or memory. However, the precise site at which the novel anxiolytics, buspirone and ipsapirone, interact to produce the antianxiety relief is still being investigated. They can act on serotoninergic autoreceptors to decrease 5-HT release. They can also activate postsynaptic 5-HT_{1A} receptor sites, resulting in decreased neuronal function (Sprouse and Aghajanian, 1988). Which of these effects is the clinically more important is still not fully understood. However, recent findings suggest that the raphe autoreceptors are a crucial site for the behavioural effects of these compounds (Olivier et al., 1989).

'Soft' results have been obtained suggesting a possible role for 5-HT_{1B}, 5-HT_{1C}, 5-HT_{1D} in mediating anxiety in animals and humans. The lack of firm findings is partly due to the absence of specific drugs. By using the available compounds, which possess mixed properties on various $5HT_1$ receptor sites, both anxiolytic and anxiogenic effects have been observed in several anxiety paradigms (Barrett, 1991).

5-HT_2 antagonists ritanserin and ketanserin, have been found to be anxiolytic both in animal tests and in humans (Leysen, 1985; Ceulemans et al., 1985). Such effects may be due to the antagonism of cortical postsynaptic 5-HT_2 receptors, again suggesting the role of cortical and limbic 5-HT terminals in anxiety states.

So far, 5-HT_2 agonists have not been widely examined in all animal models, so such results that are available appear confusing. On the other hand, it is almost impossible to differentiate the effects provoked by the interaction with 5-HT_2 receptors from those due to the activation of 5-HT_{1C} induced by these agents.

In addition to 5-HT_{1A} selective compounds, another class of 5-HT agents has been suggested as possessing novel anxiolytic properties: 5-HT_3 receptor antagonists. Initially, 5-HT_3 receptors had been extensively characterized in the peripheral nervous system: recently, the availability of ligands such as [^{3}H]-ICS 205-930 and [^{3}H]-(S) raclopride has made it possible to identify 5-HT_3 receptors in the human brain (Palacios et al., 1991). The reported distribution of 5-HT_3 binding sites in the brain is strikingly in line with the anatomical locus of the observed behavioural effects. Recent evidence suggests that 5-HT_3 antagonists display anxiolytic-like activity in several animal tests, whereas detailed clinical studies of the possible anxiolytic effects in humans have not yet been reported. The recent development of numerous potent and selective 5-HT_3 antagonists should promote further studies about the role of this receptor in the pathophysiology of human anxiety disorders. The question of whether the anxiolytic properties of the 5-HT_3 antagonists are due to the decreased 5-HT neuronal activity or are related to the influence of other specific neurotransmitter pathways (such as DA mesolimbic system) deserves further studies (Millson and Preston, 1991).

In conclusion, the available data supports the view that decreased activity of the 5-HT pathways projecting to the cortical and limbic areas may have an important involvement in the relief of anxiety states, both in animals and humans. The activation of many different mechanisms may cooperate synergically to reduce serotoninergic activity:

a) by the activation of some somatodentritic receptors in the raphe nucleus resulting in the inhibition of neuronal firing;
b) by the antagonism at 5-HT_2 receptor sites;
c) by the antagonism at 5-HT_3 receptors which affects 5-HT activity via a still unidentified mechanism.

Therefore, 5-HT anxiolytic agents represent a promising class of drugs. They may offer a new approach to the treatment of anxiety disorders with minor side effects. However, further clinical trials are needed to better assess their efficacy.

After a decade of intensive research on the structure and brain neuroanatomy of BDZ modulatory sites, our knowledge of the molecular events underlying the pharmacological effects of BDZs is such that they are now the best understood of the major neuropsychotropic drugs. It had been hoped that insights into the mechanism of action of this class of compounds would ultimately clarify the pathophysiology of anxiety. Unfortunately, compared to the fundamental advances in the understanding of the sites of action and molecular mechanisms of BDZs, the pathophysiology of anxiety states is still not completely defined. The prominent interactions of anxiolytic compounds with the omega modulatory sites of GABA operated Cl^- channels indicate that these macromolecular complexes are candidates for sites of pathology in anxiety disorders. However, it is unlikely that the $GABA_A$-omega receptor complex represents the only system involved in the pathophysiology of anxiety. The ubiquity of the GABA receptor in the brain and the well studied interactions between GABA and other systems, such as 5-HT, make this an attractive model through which anxiety symptoms may be pharmacologically influenced.

5-HT_{1A} Compounds

Buspirone

Buspirone is the first of a new class and generation of antianxiety agents called azaspirodecanadiones. It is not correlated, either pharmacologically or chemically, with BDZs or with other antianxiety agents (Baldessarini, 1996).

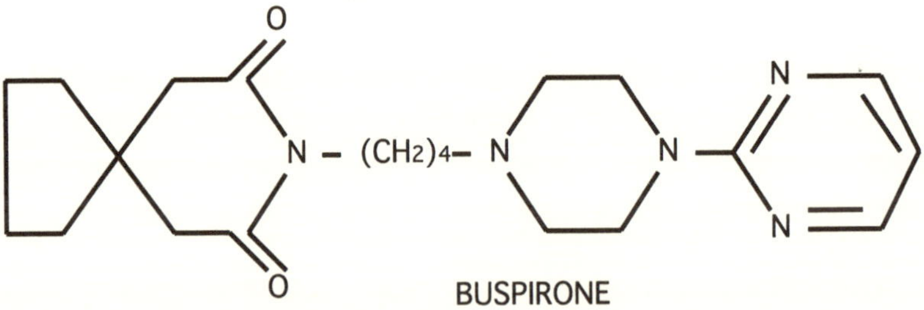

O
N – $(CH_2)_4$– N N – N N
O

BUSPIRONE

From observing the structural formula of buspirone and gepirone it may be inferred that there are some clear structural differences from BDZ anxiolytics. These lead to important differentiations between the two classes of drugs.

The compound has been selected from a sequence of psychotropic agents synthesized in the Mead Hohnson laboratories in the early 1970s. As a result of pharmacological and toxicologic evaluations, the compound proved to exert a clear antianxiety activity.

Early clinical investigations confirmed those data, which are now leading us to consider buspirone as an antianxiety drug with some interesting properties. Buspirone, in fact, does not induce the side effects which are typical of BDZs, such as sedation, muscle-relaxation and interference with CNS depressant drugs. Additionally, buspirone has no anticonvulsant activity. This particular configuration leads us to consider buspirone as a selective antianxiety drug, whose efficacy is comparable to that of BDZs and which acts by a different mechanism of action. Buspirone is well absorbed after oral administration and is subject to a rapid metabolism. Buspirone biodisponibility is directly related to the dose administered, suggesting that the therapeutic dose used does not saturate the first metabolic step.

Studies in which multiple doses of buspirone have been administered have confirmed that the pharmacokinetics of this drug is linear. Average buspirone systemic biodisponibility is around 4%, with a range between 1 and 13%. These data are in agreement with individual differences observed in patients receiving the same dose of buspirone. Food intake does not influence buspirone absorption, but biodisponibility increases 80% circa.

This phenomenum, also observed with other drugs, is probably due to food intake decreasing the first step metabolism.

In normal subjects, buspirone is rapidly eliminated. Its elimination half-life, reported in several studies, ranges between 2 and 11 hours (Gammans et al., 1985).

The main catabolic pathways of buspirone are oxidations. These processes lead to the formation of 5-hydroxy-buspirone and 1-(2-pyrimidyl)-piperazine (1-PP). Pharmacological studies indicate that 5-hydroxy-buspirone is an inactive metabolite, whereas 1-PP conserves a certain activity. This low activity together with a really high concentration of 1-PP suggest that this metabolite may contribute to the pharmacological effects obtained with buspirone (Garattini et al., 1982). However, the exact contribution of 1-PP has still to be evaluated in clinical studies. Buspirone pharmacokinetics has been evaluated in different populations. No significant differences have been observed between those subjects aged over 65 and those aged 21-40 years (Gammans et al., 1986) — whereas a similar study on BDZs reports a reduced clearance of these medications in aged people. It is therefore recommended for BDZs, but not for buspirone, to decrease the initial dose in older patients. Other studies have also shown that sex differences, as well as age differences, do not influence buspirone metabolism. Urinary and faecal excretion account for 65% and 35%, respectively, of a dose. The elimination half-life ranges from 2 to 8 hours in healthy volunteers.

As expected, since buspirone is mainly catabolized through an oxidative process, its clearance is markedly reduced in patients with impaired hepatic function. Although buspirone's side effects are limited, its administration to patients with impaired hepatic functions has to be carefully evaluated (Gammans et al., 1986). Impaired renal function causes only a modest decrement of buspirone clearance and hemodialysis does not significantly alter elimination of this drug. However, a cautious buspirone administration is recommended for patients with impaired renal function (Garattini et al., 1982). The initial starting oral dose for the therapy of generalized anxiety in adults is 5 mg three times a day. If no significant improvement is achieved after several weeks, upward adjustment of the dose is advisable.

Findings from controlled trials show a low overall incidence of side effects during treatment with buspirone. Headache, mild dizziness, paraesthesia and gastrointestinal discomfort are reported by less than 10% of subjects. About 10% of patients refer to sedation side-effects, a similar incidence to placebo (Goa and Ward, 1986).

Gepirone

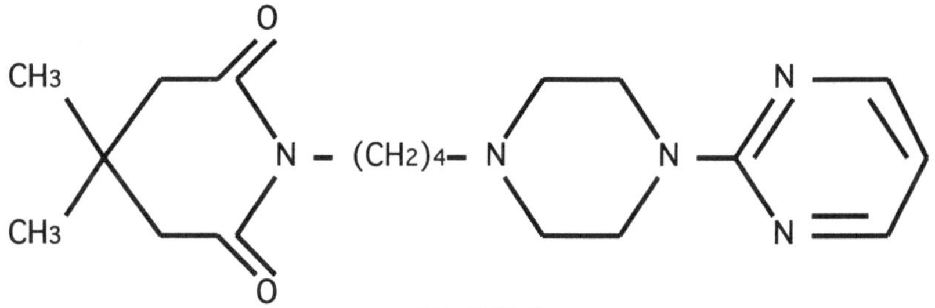

GEPIRONE

Gepirone is an analogue of buspirone that binds specifically to 5-HT_{1A} receptors and is a more complete agonist than buspirone. It is still under clinical investigation as an anxiolytic drug. It shares the pharmacological profile as buspirone and, in addition, possesses certain desirable features including greater bioavailability and greater intrinsic activity as measured by the 5-HT_{1A} adenylate cyclase assay. Gepirone falls between buspirone and the full 5-HT_{1A} agonists, such as 5-HT, in its activity in this in vitro system (Robinson, 1991).

Unlike buspirone which shows significant D_2 antagonism, gepirone is not proposed to affect dopamine mechanisms, since in binding studies it failed to show any significant affinity for the D_2 receptor. However, gepirone in rat pituitary is able to directly inhibit prolactin release, an effect blocked by haloperidol

(Nash and Meltzer, 1989). In addition, gepirone suppresses rat prolactin secretion in vivo behaving like a D_2 agonist. When given to healthy volunteers in high oral doses, gepirone increases prolactin plasma levels (Murphy et al., 1991). Whether gepirone, which is still under clinical evaluation, will prove to be therapeutically superior to buspirone can only be assessed after it has become more widely available for clinical use. Preliminary findings indicate gepirone to be as effective and potent as BDZs, but some differences have been discerned. Improvement in patients treated with gepirone seems slower than in those treated with diazepam, although they eventually catch up. This suggests that gepirone efficacy might be related to adaptive changes in the 5-HT system due to long-term 5-HT_{1A} receptor activation, or to the accumulation of a clinically active metabolite. The first proposal is supported by the recent demonstration in rats that long term administration of gepirone reduces the sensitivity of the somatodendritic 5-HT autoreceptor. This autoreceptor, which is of the 5-HT_{1A} subtype, exerts a negative feedback control on the firing activity of the central serotoninergic neurons. Like all compounds of the azopirone class, gepirone has the active metabolite 1-(2-pyrimidyl)-piperazine (1-PP), an $alpha_2$ adrenoreceptor antagonist at micromolar concentration. It is possible therefore, to speculate that alterations in noradrenergic neurotransmission might be involved, at least partially, in the psychopharmacological effects of this drug. However, since the 1-PP concentrations are in the low nanomolar range, it is unlikely that the effects of 1-PP could be of clinical value. Placebo controlled studies with gepirone (10-90 mg/day) have shown that this agent produces significant therapeutic benefit in anxiety disorders. Its benefit/risk ratio is at least as favorable as that of BDZs, and its putative lack of dependence potential should allow for a greater flexibility of treatment, as well as avoid the major problems presented by chronic BDZ users.

Ipsapirone

Ipsapirone displays high selective affinity for brain 5-HT_{1A} receptor in vitro and in vivo and possesses well-defined pharmacological properties as an 5-HT_{1A} agonist in animals. It has been found to yield a consistent pattern of effects when given to healthy volunteers in oral doses of 10-40 mg. Plasma cortisol, adrenocorticotropic hormone and growth hormone are increased, and body temperature is lowered. Plasma prolactin increased with gepirone and buspirone but not with ipsapirone. The neuroendocrine and body temperature effects of ipsapirone are antagonized by pretreatment with the 5-HT_{1A} and beta adrenergic antagonist, pindolol, and, to some extent, the non-selective 5-HT antagonist, metergoline, but not by the selective beta adrenergic antagonist, betaxolol. Ipsapirone is devoid of any dopaminergic effect.

When systemically administered in animals, ipsapirone has been found active in several models of anxiety, including the conflict, social interaction and elevated plus-maze tests, although it failed to affect the shock probe test, or block the fear-potentiated startle. Preliminary clinical results indicate that ipsapirone (10-30 mg/day; the optimal dose seems 5 mg tid) possesses anxiolytic properties in humans. It appears to offer its anxiolytic effects without the adverse effects characteristic of BDZs. In contrast to buspirone, ipsapirone clinical efficacy is not dependent on the patient's prior history of BDZ treatment. In conclusion, it appears that ipsapirone represents a viable alternative to BDZs in the treatment of anxiety disorders since it induces fewer adverse events, and is as effective without real sedation and dependence potential.

Zalospirone

Zalospirone (Wy-47,846) is a 5-HT_{1A} partial agonist with antianxiety properties in a variety of animal paradigms. Compared to buspirone and gepirone, zalospirone falls more towards the antagonist and intrinsic activity spectrum.

In binding studies, it displays the highest activity for 5-HT_{1A} receptors, 20 times greater than for D_2 or 5-HT_2 receptors. In electrophysiological investigations, zalospirone inhibits the firing rates of raphe serotoninergic neurons in a manner consistent with 5-HT_{1A} agonist. It shows antagonist properties in the behavioural 5-HT syndrome test, a 5-HT_{1A} postsynaptic-mediated response.

Zalospirone possesses anxiolytic activity in several experimental models. In mice, it antagonizes isolation-provoked aggressive behaviour in a dose dependent manner. In conflict tests and in two compartment exploration tests, zalospirone has anti-anxiety activity comparable to buspirone and BDZs.

On the basis of these pharmacological characteristics, zalospirone is being investigated as an anxiolytic agent useful in human therapy.

5-HT_3 Receptor Antagonists

The 5-HT_3 receptor is unique among monoamine receptor subtypes in forming a multi-unit ion channel analogous to the nicotinic, $GABA_A$ and glycine receptors. The binding site of the 5-HT_3 receptor class has been identified in rat brain preparations, by using several antagonists. There is evidence that 5-HT_3 receptors are present in high concentrations in discrete nuclei of lower brainstem and area postrema, in cortical and limbic structures. Studies in the human brain have also been reported to show tropisetron binding sites in the limbic system. The discovery of 5-HT_3 receptors with a peculiar distribution throughout the CNS led to increasingly intense preclinical evaluation of a possible 5-HT_3 receptor role in pathophysiology of neuro-psychic disease.

Since experimental anxiolysis can occur by suppressing 5-HT transmission in the brain, then, it is not so surprising that 5-HT_3 receptor antagonists can display antianxiety activity in animal paradigms. The 5-HT_3 antagonists, GR380327, BRL43694, ICS205-930 and raclopride all exhibit anxiolytic activity in the social interaction test in rats and the two compartment test in mice, but not in the water-lick conflict test in rats. 5-HT_3 receptor antagonists, however, appear to be inactive in the elevated plus-maze test. They also fail to show anxiolytic activity in the social interaction test, although 5-HT_3 antagonist, MDL72222 displays anxiolytic effect in this test.

Thus ondansetron, a potent and highly selective antagonist of 5-HT_3 receptors, is active in most, but not all animal models of anxiolytics. It mimics the disinhibitory properties of BDZs but lacks their sedative anticonvulsant and muscle relaxant properties. Preliminary clinical evidence suggests that it is a useful anxiolytic in humans at low doses (1 mg t.i.d.) and that in contrast to BDZs, it does not induce any psychomotor or cognitive impairment.

It has been demonstrated recently that activation of 5-HT_3 receptor results in the release of cholecystokinin (CCK) from rat brain synaptosomes. On the basis of the supposed role of CCK in anxiety, antagonism of an overactive CCK system in limbic area would be a reasonable biochemical mechanism underlaying the anxiolytic effect of 5-HT_3 receptor antagonist, and it would represent a rationale for the chemical development of both 5-HT_3 and CCK receptor antagonists as novel anxiolytic drugs (Olivier et al., 1992; Paudice and Raiteri, 1991).

5-HT_2 Agents

The involvement of 5-HT in anxiety seems to be fairly well confirmed. The confusion concerning this role is increased by the observation that anxiety often coexists with depression, a clinical condition in which the functioning of the serotoninergic mechanism is supposed to be reduced, and by the demonstration of a variety of 5-HT receptor subtypes with different functional role. Agonists and antagonists used in early investigations order to define the role of 5-HT in anxiety are now considered non specific with regard to receptor subtypes. But unfortunately, potent and selective agents are still not currently available.

5-HT_2/5-HT_{1C} receptors have been identified as postsynaptic receptors. They are coupled to phospholipase C to generate inositol phosphates and diacylglycerol as second messengers. Activation of phospholipid turnover mobilizes the intracellular Ca^{++} and activates the Ca-dependent processes.

5-HT_2 receptor stimulation results in membrane depolarization and neuronal excitation. The central 5-HT_2 sites have been identified using ^3H or iodinated antagonists with autoradiography. These investigations have demonstrated a high density of postsynaptic sites in the cortex, claustrum and olfactory tubercle followed by the caudate and nucleus accumbens, with a low density of sites in the brainstem, medulla and cerebellum. 5-HT_{1C} receptors are mostly found in the choroid plexus and show a low density in the hippocampus, the dentate gyrus and layer III of the neocortex. Also, regions which are commonly believed to be involved in the generation of anxiety (such as amygdala, septum and hippocampus) contain substantial amounts of 5-HT_2 site: this is well demonstrated in the human brain.

To investigate the precise role of 5-HT_2 receptor in anxiety states, a number of 5-HT_2 ligands have been studied. These compounds include:

- 5-HT_2 antagonists (such as altanserin, ritanserin, seganserin, ketanserin, pipamperone and MDL11939)
- ergot derivatives/mixed agonist-antagonists (metergoline, methysergide and LY-53857)
- dopamine D_2 agonist (lisuride)
- dopamine D_2 antagonists (such as ocaperidone, risperidone, spiperone, metitepine, and benperidol)
- histamine H_1 antagonists (pizotifen and cyproheptadine)
- antidepressant (mianserin)
- dopamine antagonist (SCH23390)
- gastrokinetic (cisapride).

All compounds show affinity for 5-HT_2 receptor in the nanomolar range (Leysen, 1992).

In general, all the selective 5-HT_2 antagonists show anti-anxiety effects in some animal tests. However, their activity varies considerably among the different test procedures. In rodents, limited activity or no activity at all is found in the conflict tests and in the shock probe conflict procedure.

By contrast, substantial activity is seen with different 5-HT antagonists when they are evaluated in different paradigms of open field tests and the elevated plus maze (Olivier et al., 1992). With ketanserin and ritanserin in particular, they induce a disinhibition of exploratory behavior over a wide dose range which continues after chronic treatment. An interesting property of the 5-HT_2 antagonists is that they produce down-regulation of the 5-HT_2 site in the rat after chronic administration, rather than the conventional supersensitivity observed with chronic antagonism of dopamine receptors. It is not possible to judge the value of this finding in relation to possible future clinical use. But it will be of interest to establish whether this property can be utilized to antagonize tolerance effects which can derive from chronic use of these agents (Blackshear et al., 1983; Gandolfi et al., 1983; Leysen et al., 1986; Twist et al., 1990).

Only limited data are available at present on the possible clinical anti-anxiety activity of 5-HT_2 antagonists. Preliminary results with pipamperone show a modest anxiolytic property without a confirmed dose-dependent response.

Ritanserin alone has been studied in more detail. In generalized anxiety disorder, ritanserin shows non sedative anxiolytic properties equi-effective to 5 mg of lorazepam — but it appears to be ineffective in the treatment of panic disorder. Although a growing body of evidence suggests that 5-HT_2 receptors might be implicated in some anxiety states, further clinical studies with potent and selective compounds are required.

Bibliography

Baldessarini RJ: Drugs and the treatment of psychiatric disorders. In: *Goodman and Gilman's the pharmacological basis of therapeutics.* Hardman JG, Limbird LE, Melinoff PB, Ruddon RW and Goodman Gilman A (eds.). 9th editon McGraw-Hill, New York pp. 399-430, 1996

Barrett JE Animal behaviour models in the analysis and understanding of anxiolytic drugs acting at serotonin receptors. In: *Animal Models in Psychopharmalogy.* Oliver B, Mos J and Slangen JL (eds.), Basel, Birkhauser pp. 37-52, 1991

Blackshear MA, Friedman RL and Sanders-Bush E: Acute and chronic effects of serotonin (5-HT) antagonists on serotonin binding sites. *Naunyn Schmiedebergs Arch Pharmacol* 324:125-129, 1983

Briley M and Chopin P: Serotonin in anxiety: evidence from animal models. In: *5-hydroxytryptamine in psychiatry: a spectrum of ideas.* Sandle M, Coppen A and Harnett S (eds.), Oxford Medical Publication chapter 15, pp. 177-190, 1981

Budhram P, Deacon R and Garner CR: Some putative non-sedating anxiolytics in a conditioned licking conflict. *British Journal of Pharmacology* 88:331P, 1986

Carli M, Invernizzi R, Cervo L and Samanin R: Neurochemical and behavioural studies with RU24969 in the rat. *Psychopharmacology* 94:359-364, 1988

Ceulemans DLS, Hoppenbrouwers MLJA, Gelder YG and Reyntjeus AJM: The influence of ritanserin, a serotonin antagonist, in anxiety disorders: a double-blind placebo-controlled study versus lorazepam. *Pharmacopsychiatry* 18:303-305, 1985

Colpaert FC, Meert TF, Niemegeers CJE and Janssen PAJ: Behavioral and 5-HT antagonist effect of ritanserin: a pure and selective antagonist of LSD discrimination in rat. *Psychopharmacology* 86:45-54, 1985

Costall B, Jones BJ, Kelly ME, Naylor NJ, Oakley NR, Onaive ES and Tyers MB: The effect of ondansetron (GR38032F) in rats and mice treated subchronically with diazepam. *Pharmacology Biochemistry and Behavior* 34:769-778, 1989

Costall B, Kelly ME, Tomkins DM and Tyers MB: Profile of action of diazepam and 5-HT_3 receptor antagonists on the elevated X-maze. *Journal of Psychopharmacology* 3:10P, 1989

Costall B and Naylor R: Anxiolytic potential of 5-HT_3 receptor antagonists. *Pharmacology and Toxicology* 70:157-162, 1992

Critchley MAE and Handley SL: 5-HT_2 receptor antagonists show anxiolytic activity in the Xmaze. *British Journal of Pharmacology* 89:646P, 1986
Critchley MAE and Handley SL: 5-HT_{1A} ligand effects in the x-maze anxiety test. *British Journal of Pharmacology* 92:660P, 1987
Critchley MAE and Handley SL: Dorsal raphe lesions abolish effects of 8-OH-DPAT and ipsapirone in x-maze. *British Journal of Pharmacology* 97:309P, 1989
de Montigny C and Blier P: Electrophysiological evidence for the distinct properties of presynaptic and postsynaptic 5-HT_{1A} receptors: possible clinical relevance. In: *Serotonin receptor subtypes: pharmacological significance and clinical implications*. Langer SZ, Brunello N, Racagni G and Mendlewicz J (eds.) Karger, pp. 80-88, 1992
Engel JA: Anticonflict effect of the putative serotonin agonist 8-OH-DPAT. *Psycho pharmacology* 89:S13, 1986
Eison AS, Eison MS, Stanley M and Riblet LA: Serotoninergic mechanism in the behavioural effects of buspirone and gepirone. *Pharmacology Biochemistry and Behavior* 24:701-707, 1986
Gammans RE, Mayol RF, Mackenthun AV and Sokya LF: The relationship between buspirone bioavailability and dose in healthy subjects. *Biopharm Drug Disp* 6:139-145, 1985
Gammans RE, Mayol RF and LaBudde JA: Metabolism and disposition of buspirone. *American Journal of Medicine* 80(suppl. 3B):41-51, 1986
Gandolfi O, Barbaccia ML and Costa E: Different effects of serotonin antagonist on (3H)mianserin and (3H)ketanserin recognition sites. *Life Science* 36:713-721, 1983
Garattini S, Caccia S and Mennini T: Notes on buspirone's mechanism of action. *Journal of Clinical Psychiatry* 43(section 2):19-22, 1982
Glaser T and Traber J: Buspirone: action of serotonin receptors in calf hippocampus. *European Journal of Pharmacology* 88:137-138, 1983
Goa K and Ward A: Buspirone, a preliminary review of its pharmacologycal properties and therapeutic efficacy as an anxiolytic. *Drugs* 32:114-129, 1986
Higgins GA, Jones HJ and Oakley NR: Compounds selective for the 5-HT_{1A} receptors have anxiolytic effects when injected into the dorsal raphe nucleus of the rat. *British Journal of Pharmacology* 12:658P, 1987
Howard L and Pollard GT: Effects of buspirone in the Geller-Seifter conflict test with incremental shock. *Drug Development Research* 19:37-49, 1990
Iversen SD: 5-HT and anxiety. *Neuropharmacology* 23:1553-1560, 1984
Jones BJ, Costall B, Domeney AM, Kelly ME, Naylor RJ, Oakley NR and Tyers MB: The potential anxiolytic activity of GR38032F, a 5-HT_3 receptor antagonist. *British Journal of Pharmacology* 93:985-993, 1988
Lader MH: Ondansetron in the treatment of anxiety. Presented at the 5th World Congress of Biological Psychiatry, Satellite Symposium, The role of ondansetron, a novel 5-HT_3 antagonist, in the treatment of psychiatric disorders. Florence pp. 17-19, 1991
Leysen JE: Characterization of serotonin receptor binding sites. In: *Neuro pharma cology of serotonin*. Green AR (ed.), Oxford University Press pp. 79-116, 1985
Leysen JE: 5-HT_2-receptors: location, pharmacological, pathological and physiological role. In: *Serotonin receptor subtypes: pharmacological significance and clinical implications*. Langer SZ, Brunello N, Racagni G and Mendlewicz J (eds.), Karger, pp. 31-43, 1992

Leysen JE, Van Gompel P, Gommeren W, Woestenborghs R and Janssen PAJ: Down regulation of serotonin-S2 receptor sites in rat brain by chronic treatment with the serotonin-S2 antagonists: ritanserin and septoperone. *Psychopharmacology* 88: 434-444, 1986

Mayol RF, Adamson DS, Gammans RE and LaBudde SA: Pharmacokinetics and disposition of ^{14}C-buspirone HCl after intravenous and oral dosing in man. *Clinical Pharmacology and Therapeutics* 37:210-215, 1985

Merlo-Pich and Samanin R: Disinhibitory effects of buspirone and low doses of sulpiride and haloperidol in two experimental anxiety models in rats: possible role of dopamine. *Psychopharmacology* 89:125-130, 1986

Millson DS and Preston GC: The clinical psychopharmacology of ondansetron. In: *Biological psychiatry*. Racagni G. et al. (eds.), Elsevier Science Publishers, vol 2, pp. 881-884, 1991

Moser P, Hibert M, Middlemis DN, Mir AK, Tricklebank MD and Fozard JR: Effects of MDL 73005EF in animal models predictive of anxiolityc activity. *British Journal of Pharmacology* 93:3P, 1988

Murphy DL, Lesch KP and Pigott TM: Behavioural, endocrine and other physiological effects in humans of drugs acting on the 5-HT receptor subtypes In: *Biological psychiatry*. Racagni G, Brunello N and Fukuda T (eds.), Excerpta Medica, vol. 2, pp. 697-699, 1991

Muth EA, Moyer JA, Haskins JT, Abou-Gharbia MA, Stephens RJ and Ward TJ: Zalospirone, Wy-50,324, and WAY-100,289: new serotoninergic agents with psychotherapeutic potential. *European Neuropsychopharmacology* 3:207-209, 1991

Nash JF and Meltzer HY: Effect of gepirone and ipsapirone on the stimulated and unstimulated secretion of prolactin in the rat. *Journal of Pharmacology and Experimental Therapeutics* 249:236-241, 1989

Nishikawa T and Scatton B: Inhibitory influence of GABA on central serotonergic transmission. Involvement of the habenulo-raphe pathways in the GABAergic inhibition of ascending cerebral serotonergic neurons. *Brain Research* 331:81-90, 1985

Olivier B, Mos J, Tulp M, Schipper J and Bevan P: Modulatory action of serotonin in aggressive behaviour. In: *Behavioural pharmacology of 5-HT*. Bevan P, Cools AR and Archer T (eds.), Hilsdale, Lawrence Erlbaum, pp. 89-115, 1989

Olivier B, Mos J, Tulp MTM and van der Poel AM: Animal models of anxiety and aggression in the study of serotonergic agents. In: *Serotonin receptor subtypes: pharmacological significance and clinical implications*. Langer SZ, Brunello N, Racagni G and Mendlewicz J (eds.) Karger, pp 67-79, 1992

Palacios JM, Mengod G, Pompeiano M and Waeber C: Distribution and alteration of various 5-HT receptor subtypes in control and pathological human brain. In: *Biological Psychiatry*. Racagni G et al. (eds.) Elsevier Science Publishers, vol 2, pp. 694-696, 1991

Palfreyman MG and Kehne JH: Does 5-HT have a role in anxiety and the action of anxiolytics? In: *5-Hydroxytryptamine in psychiatry: a spectrum of ideas*. Sandler M, Coppen A and Harnett S (eds.), Oxford Medical Publications, chap. 17, pp 207-227, 1991

Paudice P and Raiteri M: Cholecystokinin release mediated by 5-HT_3 receptors in rat cerebral cortex and nucleus accumbens. *British Journal of Pharmacology* 103:1790-1794, 1991

Pellow S, Johnston AL and File SE: Selective agonists and antagonists for 5-hydroxytryptamine receptor subtypes and interaction with yohimbine and FG 7142 using the elevated plus-maze test in the rat. *Journal of Pharmacology* 39:917-928, 1987

Rickels K, Weismann K and Norstand N: Buspirone and diazepam in anxiety: a controlled study. *Journal of Clinical Psychiatry* 43:81-86, 1982

Robinson DS: Buspirone in the treatment of anxiety. In: *Buspirone: mechanism and clinical aspects*. Tunnicliff G, Eison AS and Taylor DP (eds.) Academic Press, San Diego, pp. 3-17, 1991

Saner A and Pletscher A: Effect of Diazepam on cerebral 5-hydroxytryptamine synthesis. *European Journal of Pharmacology* 55:315-318, 1979

Sprouse JS and Aghajanian GK: Responses of hippocampal pyramidal cells to putative serotonin 5-HT_{1A} and 5-HT_{1B} agonists: a comparative study with dorsal raphe neurons. *Med Ann Dist Columbia* 27:707-715, 1988

Stein L, Wise CD and Belluzzi JD: Effects of benzodiazepines on central serotonergic mechanisms. In: *Mechanisms of action of benzodiazepines*. Garattini S, Mussini E and Randall LO (eds.), Raven Press, New York, pp. 299-326, 1975

Traber J and Glaser T: 5-HT_{1A} receptor-related anxiolytics. *Trends in Pharmacological Sciences* 8:432-437, 1987

Treit D: Animal models for the study of antianxiety agents: a review. *Neuroscience and Biobehavioral Reviews* 9:203-222, 1985

Twist EC, Mitchell S, Brazell C, Stahl SM and Campbell IC: 5HT2 receptor changes in rat cortex and platelets following chronic ritanserin and clorgyline administration. *Biochemical Pharmacology* 39:161-166, 1990

Wise CD, Berger BD and Stein L: Benzodiazepines: Anxiety-reducing activity by reduction of serotonin turnover in the brain. *Science* 177:180-183, 1972

Group IV
Other Compounds

Antidepressants as Anxiolytics

Over the past decade, increasing evidence has emerged that antidepressant drugs produce therapeutic benefit in some anxiety disorders, particularly when symptoms of anxiety co-exist with symptoms of depression and in the management of frequent panic attacks with or without phobia.

It is still open to question whether the effectiveness of antidepressants in situations of "mixed anxiety-depression" is due simply to a specific ability to relieve anxiety, or, conversely, to an improvement of depression, which in turn induces the relief of anxiety. However, research is providing preliminary data favouring anxiolytic effects being independent of antidepressant response. Though caution is required with regard to this issue, the efficacy of antidepressants reported also in anxiety not associated with panic, phobic, obsessive-compulsive or depressive symptoms may support the suggestion of a specific role for these agents as anxiolytics (Paykel et al., 1990).

Antidepressants prescribed as anxiolytics should be used at the recommended dose, and — unlike with BDZs — regular assumptions are essential. They take longer than BDZs to exert the antianxiety effects, and therapy for up to six weeks may be necessary to achieve significant benefits. Compliance may represent a problem, since almost two-thirds of subjects drop out from the therapy within one month because of the delay in improvement and short-term side effects. Therefore, a full explanation of both drug-benefit and drug-side effects, and demonstration of the physician's support during the first period of therapy are recommended to maximize treatment adherence.

It is possible that some antidepressants will prove to be more effective in treating particular anxiety states than others. Some clues suggest that certain pharmacological actions of antidepressants may be important for a more appropriate management of specific anxious disorders.

Drugs with secondary sedative properties, such as amitriptyline, doxepin and mianserin, are regarded as appropriate for patients with primary anxiety states — whereas all tricyclic antidepressants (TCAs) and monoamine oxidase inhibitors (MAOIs) display impressive efficacy in alleviating panic disorders (Rickels and Schweizer, 1987). Clomipramine and, to some extent, the newer serotonin selective agents are currently considered the drugs of choice with anti obsessional effects (Insel and Zohar, 1987). Certain pharmacological features of antidepressants which distinguish anti-panic, anti-anxiety, anti-obsessional properties could support the hypothesis that particular neurochemical abnormalities may be relevant to the pathophysiology of different anxiety disorders.

Bibliography

Insel TR and Zohar J.: Psychopharmacological approaches to obsessive-compulsive disorder. In: *Psycopharmacology: The third generation of progress.* Meltzer HY (ed.), Raven Press, New York, pp. 1205-1210, 1987

Paykel ES: Introduction: the role of antidepressants. In: *The anxiolytic jungle: where next?* Weatley D (ed.) John Wiley and sons Ltd. pp. 125-128, 1990

Rickels K and Schweizer EE: Current pharmacotherapy of anxiety and panic. In: *Psycopharmacology: The third generation of progress.* Meltzer HY (ed.) Raven Press, New York, pp. 1193-1203, 1987

Tricyclic Antidepressants: Pharmacological Profile

Pharmacokinetics

All the tricyclic compounds have a three-ring nucleus. Imipramine, amitriptyline and clomipramine are tertiary amines because there are two methyl groups on their nitrogen atom of the side chain. Nortriptyline, protriptyline and desipramine are secondary amines because there is only one methyl group in this position. Mianserin is a tetracyclic compound whose side chain has been cyclised to form the fourth ring. Maprotiline is tetracyclic with the same side-chain as desipramine; its fourth ring actually bridges the centre ring of the standard tricyclic nucleus.

Absorption of most heterocyclic drugs is incomplete after oral administration and there is significant first-pass metabolism. As a result of high protein binding and relatively high lipid solubility, the volume of distribution tends to be very high (ranging from 10-30 l/Kg for tertiary amines to 20-60 l/Kg for secondary amines). Tricyclics are metabolized by two major routes: transformation of the tricyclic nucleus and alteration of the aliphatic side chain. The former route involves ring hydroxylation and conjugation to form glucuronides; the latter, primary demethylation of the nitrogen. Monodemethylation of tertiary amines leads to active metabolites, secondary amines such as desipramine from imipramine and nortriptyline from amitriptyline. The ratio of methylated to demethylated forms varies widely from subject to subject. In general, the proportion of desipramine to imipramine favors the metabolite. The converse is the case with nortriptyline to its parent drug (Baldessarini, 1996).

The half-lives vary between 10-70 hours, though protriptyline and nortriptyline have longer half-lives. The pharmacokinetic parameters of various antidepressants are reported in table 1 (page 108).

Although it is recommended that tricyclics may be administered in divided doses initially, to minimize side effects, their relatively long half-lives permit the practice of a single daily dose at bed time (table 2, page 109).

However, it has to be taken into account that, at high therapeutic doses, antidepressants possess potent anticholinergic properties which, in reducing gastrointestinal tract activity, can significantly antagonize absorption. After oral administration, tricyclics yield plasma peak concentration in 2-8 hours. Plasma protein binding is typically 90% and plasma free fraction directly correlates CSF drug concentration (Rowland and Tozer, 1989). This, in addition to the extensive interindividual variability in the pharmacokinetics, makes it advisable to measure plasma concentration for the purpose of therapeutic monitoring.

Mechanism of action

The therapeutic efficacy of TCA drugs has been linked to the ability of these compounds to inhibit in vitro and in vivo, with relatively different potencies, noradrenaline, serotonin and dopamine uptake into nerve endings, thus increasing the functional amount of neurotransmitter at postsynaptic sites (table 3, page 109).

Table 1 PHARMACOKINETIC PARAMETERS OF TRICYCLIC AND TRICYCLIC-TYPE ANTIDEPRESSANTS

Drug	Vol. of Distrib. (l/Kg)	Plasma $t_{1/2}$ (h)	Protein Binding (%)	Bioavailability (%)	Active Metabolites	Therapeutic Plasma Conc. (ng/ml)
Amitriptyline	5–10	30–45	80–90	30–60	nortriptyline	80–200
Clomipramine	7–20	22–85			desmethyl	220–700
Desipramine	20–60	12–60	70–90	65		140–
Doxepin	9–31	8–22		12–45	desmethyl	30–160
Imipramine	15–30	9–24	75–95	30–75	desipramine	>180
Nortriptyline	20–57	18–90	90–95	30–80	10-hydroxy	50–150
Protriptyline	19–57	50–200	90–95	75–90		70–170
Amoxapine		8			7,8-hydroxy	
Maprotiline	15–28	20–50	85	65–75	desmethyl	200–300

Table 2 SUGGESTED ADULT DOSAGES FOR ANTIDEPRESSANTS

	Initial dose (mg/day)	Dosage range (mg/day)
Amitriptyline	25-50	75-300
Desipramine	50	75-300
Doxepin	50	50-300
Imipramine	50	75-300
Maprotiline	50	50-250
Mianserin	20	30-120
Nortriptyline	25	40-100
Protriptyline	10	50-60

Table 3 THE RELATIVE INHIBITORY POTENCIES OF ANTIDEPRESSANTS ON THE UPTAKE OF NA, 5-HT AND DA IN RAT BRAIN IN VITRO (SYNAPTOSOMES) AND IN VIVO (VARIOUS TECHNIQUES)

	In vitro			In vivo		
	NA	5-HT	DA	NA	5-HT	DA
Amineptine	-	-	++	-	-	++
Amitriptyline	++	++	-	+	(+)	-
Clomipramine	++	+++	-	++	+(+)	-
Desipramine	+++	(+)	-	+++	(+)	-
Doxepin	+	+	-	+	+	-
Imipramine	++	+(+)	-	+++	+	-
Lofepramine	+++	(+)	-	+++	(+)	-
Maprotiline	++	-	-	++	-	-
Nortriptyline	++	(+)	-	++	(+)	-
Viloxazine	+	-	-	+	-	-

+++ *very high potency;* ++ *high potency;* + *moderate potency;* — *low potency*

However, the lack of correspondence between antidepressant-induced changes in the nerve transmitter uptake and the clinical effects has focused current research on the problem of antidepressant-provoked adaptive modification in monoamine and other neurotransmitter receptor systems.

There is preclinical evidence that all antidepressants with diverse chemical structures and different acute effects on central neurotransmission, possess the property to decrease the functional activity of postsynaptic beta adrenoceptors and to enhance the activity of 5-HT_2 receptor sites in the limbic regions of brain. Antidepressants have also been found to potentiate responses to alpha-adrenergic, dopaminergic and, to some extent, GABAergic stimulation. The time-course of these changes is similar to the time-course of therapeutic actions of antidepressants (Leonard, 1989).

Side effects

The side effects of tricyclics are often more than a minor or a transient nuisance (table 4), and involve many systems of the body.

Due to their antimuscarinic effects, these compounds may significantly affect the activity of the cardiovascular system. These effects may become lethal in the case of overdose. The most common cardiac side effects are postural hypotension and a mild sinus tachycardia. Moreover, the effect of other cardiac depressant drugs may be augmented by TCAs. Considerable precaution should be exercised in using these compounds in patients with cardiac disease (Glassman et al., 1987).

Anticholinergic activity of these compounds may also induce a dry mouth, a metallic or sour taste, epigastric distress, blurred vision, dizziness, constipation and urinary retention. Quite common side effects are excessive sweating and weight gain. Older patients suffer more of all these side effects from TCAs.

Among their other side effects caused by their interaction at CNS level, tremor occurs in almost 10% of patients receiving these drugs. TCAs may also induce weakness and fatigue due to their central effects. An increased risk of tonic-clonic seizures is associated with the use of these compounds.

The interaction of TCAs with other drugs may originate serious clinical problems. Drugs such as phenytoin, phenylbutazone, aspirin, aminopyrine, scopolamine, and phenothiazines can reduce the binding of TCAs to plasma proteins. The effect of TCAs may also be potentiated by interference, exerted by other drugs, on their metabolism at the hepatic level. Conversely, an increased metabolism of TCAs may be induced by drugs such as barbiturates and other sedatives, oral contraceptives or cigarette smoking which are responsible for induction of the microsomal enzyme system (BDZs lack this effect). Due to their anticholinergic effect, it is important to check carefully the use of TCAs simultaneously with antipsychotic drugs, antiparkinsonian agents and other compounds with anticholinergic activity.

Continued administration of these compounds may induce tolerance to the anticholinergic effects, but only occasionally is there physical dependence.

Table 4 SIDE EFFECTS OF ANTIDEPRESSANTS

Type	Minor, early	Major
Sedation	Lassitude, fatigue	Sleepiness, impaired counsciousness with alcohol and other drugs
Sympathomimetic	Tachycardia, tremor, sweating	Agitation, insomnia, aggravation of psychosis
Antimuscarinic	Blurred vision, constipation, urinary hesitancy, fuzzy thinking	Aggravation of glaucoma, paralytic ileus, urinary retention, delirium
Cardiovascular	Orthostatic hypotension, electrocardiographic abnormalities	Delayed cardiac conduction, arrhytmias, cardiomyopathy, sudden death
Psychiatric	Confusion	Central antimuscarinic syndrome, withdrawal
Neurologic	Tremor, paresthesias, electroencephalographic alterations	Seizures, neuropathy
Allergic/toxic	/	Cholestatic jaundice, agranulocytosis
Metabolic/endocrine	Weight gain, sexual disturbances	Gynecomastia, amenorrhea
Birth defects	/	Uncertain
Hematologic	/	Hemolytic anemia (nomifensine)

To avoid a withdrawal syndrome, it is opportune to gradually suspend the administration over a period of a week or even more (Baldessarini, 1996).

Bibliography

Baldessarini RJ: Drugs and the treatment of psychiatric disorders. In: *Goodman and Gilman's the pharmacological basis of therapeutics*. Hardman JG, Limbird LE, Molinoff PB, Ruddon RW and Goodman Gilman A (eds.) 9th edition, McGraw-Hill, New York, pp. 399-430, 1996

Glassman AH, Roose SP, et al.: Cardiovascular effects of tricyclic antidepressants. In: *Psycopharmacology: The third generation of progress*. Meltzer HY (ed.), Raven Press, New York, pp. 1437-1442, 1987

Leonard BE: The amine hypothesis of depression: a reassessment. In: *Biochemical and pharmacological aspects of depression.* Tipton KF and Youdim MBH (eds.), Taylor and Francis, London, 1989

Rowland M and Tozer TN: *Clinical pharmacokinetics: concepts and applications.* Second edition. Lea and Febiger, Philadelphia, 1989

Selective Serotonin Reuptake Inhibitors

In addition to their therapeutic value in the treatment of mild and severe depression, selective 5-HT reuptake inhibitors (SSRIs) have also been shown to have a role in treating anxiety disorders (Feighner and Boyer, 1991) — for two main reasons:

1) SSRIs are more effective than noradrenergic reuptake inhibitors for the management of anxiety
2) SSRIs may prove to be better tolerated than TCAs.

Many clinical trials have demonstrated the effectiveness of these compounds in panic and obsessive-compulsive disorders, whereas there are still few data supporting the view that the use of SSRI may be appropriate in alleviating symptoms in generalized anxiety.

Paradoxically, with some drugs which selectively block 5-HT reuptake a transient increase in anxious simptomatology, including agitation, may be observed at the beginning of treatment. If stimulatory side effects do occur, the dose should be decreased until the symptoms subside, though they usually resolve themselves if treatment continues (table 5).

Table 5 SUGGESTED ADULT DOSAGES FOR SSRIs

	Initial dose (mg/day)	Dosage range (mg/day)
Citalopram	20	40-60
Fluoxetine	20	20-80
Fluvoxamine	50	100-300
Paroxetine	20	20-50
Sertraline	50	100-200

Pharmacological profile

Fluoxetine, fluvoxamine, paroxetine and sertraline act through the potent and selective inhibition of the reuptake of the neurotransmitter 5-HT in the brain neurons. By inhibiting the active transport mechanism of serotonin, they are believed to exert a therapeutic effect through an increased concentration of the neurotransmitter at the synaptic cleft, thereby enhancing serotoninergic transmission.

Their relative selectivity and potency for 5-HT vs catecholamine reuptake in rat brain synaptosome preparations in vitro are shown in table 6.

Table 6 POTENCY OF INHIBITION OF [^{3}H]-MONOAMINE UPTAKE INTO RAT SYNAPTOSOMES

	Ki (nM)		
	5-HT	NA	DA
Paroxetine	1.11	349	2000
Sertraline	7.4	1410	230
Fluoxetine	25	500	4200
Fluvoxamine	6.3	1100	>10000
Clomipramine	7.5	95	9100
Amitripyline	88	79	4300
Imipramine	100	64	8500

A concentration higher than used with 5-HT is needed to inhibit the reuptake of catecholamines paroxetine is the most selective. The selectivity and potency of these molecules as 5-HT reuptake blockers in vivo after oral administration to rodents have been reported by several investigations.

It is now well established that the in vivo metabolism of TCAs generates compounds with pharmacological properties different from the parent molecule in terms of potency and/or selectivity. In the case of the tertiary tricyclics, metabolism results in moieties that are much more potent in inhibiting noradrenaline uptake than the parent molecule.

The steady-state plasma levels of the metabolites are at least as great as the parent molecule's; thus the metabolites are likely to contribute to the clinical profile of the drug.

Of the SSRIs, fluoxetine and sertraline are metabolized to pharmacologically active products.

The metabolism of fluoxetine to nor-fluoxetine results in a compound with similar transmitter uptake blocking properties to the parent drug, but with an elimination half-life longer than fluoxetine (fluoxetine half-life ranges between 1.1 and 9.2 days with a mean value of 3.6 days, whereas norfluoxetine half-life varies between 3.2 and 9.8 days with a mean value of 6.1 days). The degradation of sertraline to nor-sertraline generates a compound that is less potent than sertraline in inhibiting both 5-HT and noradrenaline uptake.

Like fluoxetine, the active metabolite of sertraline has a half-life 2 or 3 times longer than the parent drug. However, the metabolites of both paroxetine and fluvoxamine are reported as inactive on the amine uptake process.

SSRIs are devoid of significant affinity for neurotransmitter receptors, including alpha$_1$, alpha$_2$ beta adrenoceptors, dopamine, histamine H_1, 5-HT, muscarinic, GABA and opiate receptors.

Electrophysiological evidence shows that these compounds desensitise the terminal 5-HT autoreceptors on serotoninergic pathways. They do not share this action at the autoreceptors with tricyclics, as these agents sensitise postsynaptic 5-HT receptors. SSRIs leave the sensitivity of postsynaptic receptor sites unchanged. As a result, it is suggested that both tricyclics and SSRIs potentiate postsynaptic serotoninergic function with different mechanisms.

It is still unclear whether this difference in the mechanism of action of these drugs indicates differences in the therapeutic profiles (Rudorfer and Potter, 1989; Johnson, 1991; Kaye et al., 1989; Lamberger et al., 1985; Claasen, 1983; Doogan and Gunn, 1990; Johnson, 1992).

Pharmacokinetics

TCAs are similar in structure, but exert a multitude of different actions. The SSRIs are the opposite — chemically different, but pharmacologically similar. All are well absorbed orally and exhibit an extensive first-pass extraction in the liver. They are widely distributed in the body tissues and highly bound to plasma proteins. Body clearance of these drugs is accomplished almost entirely by hepatic metabolism. The metabolism of paroxetine proceeds via a well-known pathway of oxidation, followed by methylation and finally conjugation with glucuronide or sulphate. The majority of the dose is eliminated in the urine as these conjugates. Fluoxetine is eliminated by metabolism, partly to its N-demethylated metabolite nor-fluoxetine. The renal clearance of unchanged fluoxetine accounted for less than 5% of a single 40 mg oral dose. While norfluoxetine is the predominant metabolite in plasma, renal clearance of unchanged nor-fluoxetine is also minimal — less than 10% of its total clearance. Other metabolic compounds are conjugates of fluoxetine and nor-fluoxetine and hippuric acid. The metabolic pattern of fluvoxamine generates at least 32 different metabolic products. Two of the identified metabolites have been found to possess little or no effect on aminergic reuptake process and can be considered to be inactive at therapeutic concentrations; this is likely to be true for the other derivatives as well. Sertraline is metabolized by oxidation of the methoxy group to desmethylsertraline. The desmethyl metabolite, present in the plasma at concentrations ranging between 66 and 250% of the parent drug, is active to a lesser extent in inhibiting 5-HT uptake. With the exception of fluoxetine, which has an elimination half-life of 2 to 3 days, the other drugs have half-lives of about 1 day. Paroxetine and fluvoxamine achieve steady-state within 4 to 14 days of chronic dosing, whereas for fluoxetine, and particularly nor-fluoxetine, steady-state is not reached for weeks. The pharmacokinetics of these agents are characterized by marked intersubject variability (table 7).

Table 7 MEAN PHARMACOKINETIC PARAMETER OF SSRIs IN MAN

Parameter	Citalopram	Fluoxctine	Fluvoxamine	Paroxetine	Sertraline
Time of peak plasma concentration (h)	3	4-7.5	2-8	3-7	5-10
Elimination half-life (h)	35	25-220	15	25	26
Protein binding (%)	80	45	75	95	> 95
Time for steady-state plasma concentration (days)		14-28	10	4-15	
Volume of distribution (l/Kg)	9-17	25	> 6	12	24

Adverse effects

In general, SSRIs are well tolerated. The main adverse effects occurring with greater frequency than with placebo are nausea and vomiting, diarrhea, anorexia, tremor and agitation. It is important to note that these drugs cause significantly fewer anticholinergic side effects, and sometimes none at all.

SSRIs have caused small, but statistically significant, temporary reductions in body weight, in contrast to the increases frequently associated with the tricyclics antidepressants. SSRIs may produce a clinically unimportant slight reduction in heart rate.

In view of the absence of a sedative action, cardiotoxicity, anticholinergic effects and impairment of psychomotor performance, these drugs are highly suitable for administration to the elderly.

Because of the mode of SSRIs metabolism, patients with hepatic or renal insufficiency should be started on a low dosage and monitored carefully.

Convulsion may occur under treatment with SSRIs, and they should be avoided in patients with a history of epilepsy.

Bibliography

Claasen V: Review of the animal pharmacology of fluvoxamine. *British Journal of Clinical Pharmacology* 15:349S-355S, 1983

Doogan DP and Gunn KP: Sertraline, a novel antidepressant. In: *Antidepressants: 30 years on*. Leonard B and Spencer P (eds.), CNS Clinical Neuroscience, London, pp. 372-382, 1990

Feighner JP and Boyer WF (eds.): *Selective serotonin re-uptake inhibitors*. John Wiley and Sons, Chichester, 1991

Johnson AM: The comparative pharmacological properties of selective serotonin reuptake inhibitors in animals. In: *Perspectives in Psychiatry Vol 1, Selective serotonin re-uptake inhibitors*. Feighner JP and Boyer WF (eds.), John Wiley and Sons, Chichester, pp. 37-70, 1991

Johnson AM: Paroxetine: a pharmacological review. *International Clinical Psychopharmacology* 6 (Suppl. 4):15-24, 1992

Kaye CM, Haddock RE, Langley PF, et al.: A review of the metabolism and pharmacokinetics of paroxetine in man. *Acta Psychiatrica Scandinavica*, 80 (Suppl. 350):65-70, 1989

Lamberger L, Bergstrom RF, Wolen RL et al.: Fluoxetine: clinical pharmacology and physiological disposition. *Journal of Clinical Psychiatry* 46:14-19, 1985

Rudorfer MV and Potter WZ: Antidepressants: a comparative review of the clinical pharmacology and therapeutic use of the "newer" versus the "older" drugs. *Drugs* 37:713-738, 1989

Monoamine Oxidase Inhibitors

Monoamine oxidase inhibitors (MAOIs) have also been used in the treatment of anxiety disorders. These compounds were the first drugs to be employed in the pharmacotherapy of conditions where panic attacks and phobic symptoms are leading features.

Phenelzine has been the most studied MAOI, and the results indicate that it is undoubtedly superior to placebo, and at least as efficacious as imipramine in ameliorating panic attacks with or without agoraphobia (Sheehan et al., 1980) (Tyrer and Shawcross, 1988). The new MAOIs, the reversible monoamino oxidase-A (MAO-A) inhibitors, have been recently reported to be beneficial in blocking attacks and reducing anxiety in panic disorder suffers. These novel compounds may therefore be considered as an effective alternative, with a better pharmacological profile than standard MAOIs (Bakish, 1992). Over time, it is becoming apparent that MAOIs may represent the most powerful of the antipanic medications, as they possess greater anxiolytic effects than tricyclics. The data presently available suggest that MAOIs, TCAs and the high potency BDZs are all valuable in improving panic disorders — with a hierarchy of effectiveness in which antidepressants are believed to work better than BDZs.

MAOIs, particularly phenelzine, have also been employed in phobic anxiety.

Studies of mixed agoraphobic and social phobic patients have shown that phenelzine is more effective than placebo in both groups (Tyrer et al., 1973), whereas there is no evidence that pharmacotherapy with tricyclics or MAOIs is of any value in the treatment of simple phobia. At present, the availability of selective and reversible inhibitors of the monoamino oxidase (MAO), which seem to posses efficacy similar to phenelzine without the risks and side effects, is very promising (Liebowitz, 1992).

MAOIs have not been formally tested in the treatment of generalized anxiety disorder (GAD).

The most convincing evidence of the effectiveness of MAOIs in GAD derives from clinical trials performed in a populations of mixed anxiety-depression patients. These studies found that phenelzine at 60 mg/day is more effective than placebo and amitriptyline in alleviating anxiety symptoms, and that phenelzine helps anxiety better than depression (Ravaris et al., 1976; Paykel et al, 1982).

The acceptance that MAOIs cover a much wider therapeutic field than that originally assigned is of considerable importance. The therapeutic introduction of reversible MAO-A inhibitors, which represent the major advance in the pharmacology of this class of drugs in recent years, is likely to result in a wider prescription of these compounds in anxiety.

Pharmacological profile

The pharmacological effects of MAOIs are related to their capacity to block oxidative deamination of naturally occurring monoamines. These drugs block not only MAO but also other enzymes and may interfere with the hepatic metabolism of many drugs. They are analogous to TCAs in that although the maximum MAO inhibition is reached in a few days, the clinical therapeutic effect is achieved after two or three weeks of treatment. The most serious toxic effect of MAOIs is the hypertensive crisis. Inhibition of MAO enzymes in the liver by administration of MAOIs blocks the normal metabolism of tyramine and other amines ingested with food or produced by bacteria in the gut. These amines may then induce the release of catecholamines which are present, in augmented concentration, in nerve terminals and the adrenal medulla, and cause the hypertensive crisis. In certain instances, this may be lethal. The occurrence of this toxic effect was the main reason why the use of MAOIs was limited. However, it now appears that the risk of death caused by an improvised hypertensive crisis related to ingestion of tyramine-rich food has been exaggerated.

The potential toxicity of MAOIs involves mainly the liver, the brain and the cardiovascular system. Their hepatotoxicity does not seem to correlate to the dosage and duration of treatment. Although the incidence of this kind of toxicity is low, when it does occur the damage, to the hepatic parenchyma, is serious. An excessive central stimulation (consisting of tremor, insomnia and hyperhidrosis and rarely of hallucination, confusion and convulsions) and orthostatic hypotension may occur with the use of MAOIs. A variety of other less serious side effects has also been reported.

In the last few years, there has been increasing interest in this class of drugs because of the marked progress achieved in understanding the enzymatic mechanism and the structure of the MAO enzyme and the discovery of new, selective and reversible inhibitors.

Two types of MAO, denominated MAO-A and MAO-B, are present in the CNS and in the peripheral organs in mammals. Human placenta and intestine contain mainly MAO-A, while blood platelets contain MAO-B. Both enzymes are present in the liver and brain. In the brain, MAO-B is prevalent. The substrate and the inhibitor selectivity of MAO-A and MAO-B are not absolute but concentration dependent. In the human brain, the preferred substrate for MAO-A is 5-HT, while beta-phenylethylamine is a MAO-B substrate. Both enzymes catabolize DA, tyramine, NE and tryptamine.

Phenelzine as iproniazide, isocarboxazide, nialamid and tranylcypromine are irreversible nonselective MAOIs. Because the MAO inhibition by MAOIs is irreversible, it takes approximately 2 weeks after their discontinuation before the body has synthesized enough new MAO to restore its baseline concentrations.

Phenelzine is rapidly adsorbed, with maximum concentration occurring between 2 and 4 hours after administration. Plasma elimination half-lives range from 1.5 to 4 hours. After 6 to 8 weeks of administration plasma, phenelzine concentration increases compared to initial treatment value. The drug, or its metabolites, probably inhibit its own metabolism. Due to the similarity of phenelzine with other drugs, such as isoniazid, it was thought that phenelzine was metabolized by acetylation. However, contrasting findings questioned acetylation as a predominant metabolic process for phenelzine. The metabolic pathways of phenelzine for which there is supporting evidence are:

a) phenelzine is a substrate for MAO, forming phenylacetic acid
b) the drug can be metabolized to beta-phenylethylamine, a MAO substrate
c) a third potential metabolic pathway is a ring hydroxylation.

There is no definitive rationale for choosing one classical MAOI over an other, except that tranylcypromine appears to be the most activating of the drugs. Table 8 shows the usual dose range advised in adults.

Predictable dangerous interactions occur between the MAOIs and any amine precursors, or directly or indirectly acting sympathomimetics.

MAOIs interfere with the metabolism of many different classes of drugs that may be given concurrently. They potentiate the actions of general anaesthetics, antihistamines, centrally acting analgesic, sedatives and anticholinergic drugs. Dangerous interactions can occur with tricyclic. Changing a patient from one MAOI to another, or to a TCA, requires a wash-out of at least 15 days to avoid a possibility of a drug interaction.

With the new non TCAs, a longer wash-out period is recommended -not less than 4 weeks for patients on fluoxetine because of the long life of the active metabolite, nor-fluoxetine.

A series of selective inhibitors of MAO-A has been developed recently, whose actions are rapidly reversible, so that they have much less ability to provoke the unwanted interference with foods drugs than the non selective MAOIs.

Moclobemide, broforamine and toloxatone represent compounds of much interest among newly discovered MAOIs. They are not only selective MAO-A inhibitors in humans, but are also reversible and short acting. This explains why moclobemide, broforamine and toloxatone show less interaction with ingested tyramine compared with previous MAO inhibitors. A high concentration of ingested tyramine, which is mainly degraded by MAO-A in the intestine, can displace a reversible short acting inhibitor from the intestinal MAO-A and can be made inactive by the enzyme. These peculiar characteristics of reversible inhibitors of MAO-A and their good tolerability make these compounds promising drugs in the treatment of depression as well as phobic and panic disorders.

Table 8 SUGGESTED ADULT DOSES FOR SOME NOT REVERSIBLE MAOIs

MAOI	Usual Daily Dose (mg)	Extreme Daily Dose * (mg)
Tranylcypromine	20-30	10-40
Isocarboxazide	10-30	10-30
Phenelzine	15-30	15-90

** Extreme doses are for very young and elderly subjects at the low end and for hospitalized patients at the high end.*

The new MAOIs do not have any specific biochemical and pharmacological actions. Their effect on MAO-A is thought to be the most likely mechanism underlaying their therapeutic properties. In brain and many other tissues, they increase the concentrations of the preferential substrates of MAO-A, NA and 5-HT. In parallel, CSF, plasma and urinary concentrations of NA metabolite, 3-methoxy-4-hydroxyphenylglycol (MHPG), are reduced. Table 9 summarizes the pharmacokinetics of both brofaromine and moclobemide.

Table 9 PHARMACOKINETICS OF BROFAROMINE AND MOCLOBEMIDE

Drug	t 1/2 (hours)	F (%)	Vol distr (l/kg)	CL TOT (ml/min)	Protein binding (%)
Moclobemide	1.6	56-90	0.6-1.6	657	50
Brofaromine	14-16	87	3.8	182	98

There are major differences in the kinetics of the two compounds. Brofaromine is largely metabolized by the liver to the inactive O-desmethyl metabolite. Moclobemide undergoes a large first-pass metabolism. It is almost completely metabolized by at least four pathways to inactive metabolites. The bioavailability (F) of a single oral dose of 100 mg is 56%. It increases dose dependently to 90% with repeated administration of 150 mg t.i.d. This suggests a saturable hepatic metabolism.

Reversible MAO-A inhibitors are suggested to display a spectrum of clinical efficacy comparable with classical non reversible MAOIs although the newer MAOIs have not been tested sufficiently for their place in therapeutics to be established.

Effective dosage is quite variable. Brofaromine is given in doses from 50 mg/day to 50 mg t.i.d. Moclobemide therapeutic dosage ranges from 100 mg t.i.d. to 200 mg t.i.d. There is no correlation between plasma concentration and response. Routine monitoring of the concentrations seems to be unnecessary.

Bibliography

Bakish D: Reversible Monoaminooxidase A inhibitors in panic attacks. *Clinical Neuropharmacology* 15:432-433, 1992

Katzung BG: *Basic and clinical pharmacology*. Katzung BG (ed.), Apleton and Lange Publisher, Los Angeles, 1987

Liebowitz MR: Reversible MAO inhibitors in social phobia, bulimia and other disorders. *Clinical Neuropharmacology* suppl. 1:434-435, 1992

Paykel SE, Rowan PR, Parker RR and Bath AV: Response to phenelzine and amitriptyline in subtypes of neurotic depression. *Archives of General Psychiatry* 39:1041-1049, 1982

Ravaris CL, Nies A, Robinson DS, Ives JO and Bartlett D: A multiple dose controlled study of phenelzine in depressive-anxiety states. *Archives of General Psychiatry* 33:347-350, 1976

Sheehan DV, Ballenger JC and Jacobsen G: Treatment of endogenous anxiety with phobic, hysterical, and hypochondriacal symptoms. *Archives of General Psychiatry* 37:51-59, 1980

Tyrer P, Candy J and Kelly D: A study of the clinical effects of phenelzine and placebo in the treatment of phobic anxiety. *Psychopharmacologia* 32:237-254, 1973

Tyrer P and Shawcross C: Monoamine oxidase inhibitors in anxiety disorders. *Journal of Psychiatry Research* 22 (suppl. 1):87-98, 1988

Alpha$_2$ Adrenoreceptor Agonist: Clonidine

Central noradrenergic disregulation has been implicated in the pathogenesis of anxiety (Uhole et al., 1984). A substantial body of preclinical data points toward involvement of the locus coeruleus (LC), the major noradrenaline-containing nucleus in the brain, in the mediation of anxiety, although this view is still not fully accepted, and remains controversial (Redmond jr., 1979).

In laboratory animals the greatest change in the firing of LC neurones occurs on the presentation of novel and challenging stimuli, and anxiety states may be associated with chronic overactivity of the brain noradrenergic neurones and increased sensitivity of the LC to adverse stimuli (Rasmussen et al., 1986; Redmond, 1979).

Clonidine, a relatively selective alpha$_2$ agonist, attenuates central noradrenergic activity by reducing firing of LC neurones and inhibits behavioral responses induced by LC activation. Due to this property, clonidine arouses stimulates interest for its possible therapeutic effect in the treatment of anxiety disorders (Redmond, 1982). Initial clinical application has been in the treatment of opiate withdrawal, where anxiety is a well known and prominent feature (Gold et al., 1978). Its successful use in ameliorating symptoms in this syndrome, in which noradrenergic hyperactivity is believed to be implicated as the underlaying mechanism, has supported the view about the anxiolytic role for clonidine.

However, clonidine's anxiolytic property was questioned after it appeared to possesses only a weak efficacy in affecting the symptoms of a broad spectrum of anxiety states. To date, results from most controlled studies indicate that clonidine's anxiolytic effect is modest and generally transient, since benefits wane with time as tolerance develops (Rickels and Schweirer, 1987).

Tolerance to the anxiolytic effect of chronic treatment has been postulated to be due to the desensitation of LC $alpha_2$ autoreceptors.

The evidence is therefore convincing that clonidine possesses only limited indications, since it is able, through its relatively specific action on noradrenergic function, to simply improve anxiety symptoms in conditions where noradrenergic overactivity is the primary component of the syndrome. Conversely the failure of clonidine to be a consistently effective treatment of anxiety states implies that noradrenergic disturbances do not represent the prominent neurochemical abnormality in human anxiety, but dysfunctions of a number of other neurotransmitter systems, including GABA, 5-HT and adenosine, have to be considered important factors.

Pharmacological profile

Clonidine is well absorbed after oral administration and peak plasma concentrations are observed in 1-3 hours. Its bioavailability averages 85% and the half-life is 8-12 hours. About half of the drug is eliminated unchanged in the urine. Due to its relatively short half-life, clonidine has to be administered twice daily to maintain effective blood concentrations. Therapeutic doses are commonly between 5-10 mg/Kg/day. The pattern of adverse effect includes dry mouth, while sedation occurs in at least 50% of patients — requiring, in certain cases, discontinuation of the drug. However, these centrally mediated effects may diminish with time as tolerance appears. Sexual complaints may be also reported. The drug should not be prescribed to patients which are at risk of depression and should be discontinued if depression emerges under treatment. Withdrawal effects follow abrupt discontinuation and severe hypertensive crises, mediated by sympathetic overactivity, may occur.

Bibliography

Gold MS, Redmond DE jr and Kleber HD: Clonidine in opiate withdrawal. *Lancet* 1:929, 1978

Rasmussen K, Morilak DA and Jacobs BL: Single unit activity of locus coeruleus in the freely moving cat. I During naturalistic behaviours and response to simple and complex stimuli. *Brain Research* 371:324-34, 1986

Redmond DE jr: New and old evidence for the involvement of a brain norepinephrine system in anxiety. In: *The Pharmacology and treatment of anxiety*. Fann WE (ed.), Jamaica NY Spectrum Publishers Inc., pp. 153-203, 1979

Redmond DE: New and old evidence for the involvement of a brain norepinephrine system in anxiety. In: *Phenomenology and treatment of anxiety*. Fann WE, Karacan I, Pokorny AD, et al. (eds.), SP Medical and Scientific Books, New York, 1979

Redmond DE: Does clonidine alter anxiety in humans? *Trends in Pharmacological Sciences* 3:477-480, 1982

Rickels K and Schweirer EE: *Current pharmacotherapy of anxiety in psychopharmacology: the third generation of progress*. Meltzer HY (ed.), pp. 1193-1204, 1987
Uhole T, Boulenger JP, Post RM et al.: Fear and anxiety: relationship to noradrenergic function. *Psychopatology* 17 (suppl. 3):8-23, 1984

Beta-Blockers

Many somatic symptoms of anxiety involve overactivity of the beta-adrenergic system. Pharmacologic blockade of this hyperactivity might be expected to be of benefit in reducing peripheral manifestations of anxiety, such as tachycardia, tremor and sweating. Results from several clinical trials over the past years have been consistent with this assumption.

Furthermore, the ability of beta-blockers — which penetrate into the brain — to antagonize some features of anxiety in a number of animal paradigms, has suggested the possibility that these drugs might also be effective in alleviating the psychic component of anxiety (Bainbridge and Greenwood, 1971). However, despite this premise, many studies demonstrate the lack of any significant effect of beta-blockers in influencing psychological symptoms of anxiety, such as worry, tension and fear. At first regarded as a promising therapeutic alternative to BDZs, beta-blockers now appear inadequate to fully replace BDZs in the treatment of anxiety — since they are effective only in the control of somatic manifestation, mainly when induced as a response to stressful situations, and are unable to significantly improve the psychological complaints (Noyes, 1992).

Propanolol and similar beta-receptor antagonists are therefore indicated for patients with predominantly somatic symptoms, and this may in turn prevent the onset of worry and fear. The combination of a BDZ with a beta-blocker could produce more positive results than the BDZ alone (Noyes, 1984). For instance, it has been found that a mixture of alprazolam and propranolol in panic disorder, titrating the dose of each with respect to the proportion of psychic and somatic anxiety symptoms, may be more effective than using either drug alone. This would suggest more an adjunctive than a primary therapeutic role for beta-blockers in the treatment of anxiety (Lader, 1988).

Pharmacological profile

Drugs in this category share the common feature of antagonizing the effect of catecholamines at beta-adrenoreceptors.

Beta-blocking drugs occupy beta-receptor and competitively reduce receptor occupancy by catecholamines and other beta-agonists.

Most beta-blockers in clinical use are pure antagonists and the occupancy of a beta-receptor by such a drug does not activate the receptor. However, some beta-blockers cause partial activation, albeit less than the full agonists, epinephrine and norepinephrine. Another major difference among beta-antagonists is linked to their different affinities at $beta_1$ and $beta_2$ receptors. Some of these agents display a higher affinity for $beta_1$ than for $beta_2$ receptors, and this selectivity is believed to possess clinical implications. The last important differences among beta-blockers relate to their pharmacokinetic properties.

For the most part, this class of drugs is well absorbed after oral ingestion yielding plasma peak concentration after 1-3 hours.

Table 10 shows the pharmacokinetic characteristics of several beta receptor-blocking agents.

Table 10 PHARMACOKINETIC PARAMETERS OF SOME BETA-BLOCKERS

	Selectivity	Partial agonist activity	Elimination half-life (hours)	Approximate bioavailability (%)
Acebutolol	$Beta_1$	Yes	3-4	50
Atenolol	$Beta_1$	No	6-9	40
Metoprolol	$Beta_1$	No	3-4	50
Pindolol	None	Yes	3-4	90
Propranolol	None	No	3.5-6	30*
Timolol	None	No	4-5	50

** Bioavailability is dose-dependent*

A variety of unwanted effects have been reported for beta-antagonists. CNS effects include sedation, sleep disturbances and depression. It has been claimed that beta receptor antagonists with low lipid solubility will have a lower incidence of neurological side effects, compared to compounds with higher lipid solubility. The major adverse effects of beta receptor antagonists relate to the predictable pharmacological consequences of beta blockade. $Beta_2$ receptor blockade associated with the use of nonselective agents commonly causes worsening of pre-existing asthma and beta blockers should not be prescribed to patients with any history of asthma. Similarly, beta receptor blockade depresses myocardial contractility and excitability. In patients with abnormal myocardial function considerable caution must be exercised in using these drugs. A very small dose of beta antagonist, eg. 20 mg of propranolol, as a bed dose, should be administered to detect individual susceptibility of the patient as shown by bradycardia (below 60 beat/min at rest).

If no particular sensitivity is found, 20 mg of propranolol four time a day may be the starting dose. It will be increased to 40 mg 4 times a day over 2 weeks period.

The resting heart rate should be monitored and regarded as the end-point: posologie should be maintained at that required to permit a normal pulse rate.

To minimize side-effects, it is not useful to increase the dose beyond 160 mg/day. At this dose, propranolol is believed to moderate somatic manifestation of anxiety by acting peripherally rather than centrally, since experimental evidence failed to show a CNS effect of single doses of propranolol up to 120 mg/day.

Moreover, it would be inadvisable to use beta antagonists in insulin-dependent diabetics, if reasonable alternatives are available.

Finally, the possible hazards of abruptly discontinuing beta-blockers after prolonged treatment must be kept in mind. Interruption may induce a withdrawal syndrome that is reminiscent of sympathetic hyperactivity. Therefore, prudence suggests the gradual tapering, rather than abrupt interruption of the administration, when the therapy is discontinued. The mechanism underlaying this effect is still unknown, but hyperactivity or up-regulation of the number of beta receptors might be involved.

Bibliography

Bainbridge JG and Greenwood DT: Tranquilizing effects of propanolol in rats. *International Journal of Neuropharmacology* 10:453, 1971

Lader M: Beta-adrenoreceptor antagonist in neuropsychiatry: an update. *Journal of Clinical Psychiatry* 49:213-223, 1988

Noyes R: Beta-blocking drugs and anxiety. *Psychosomatics* 23:155, 1992

Noyes R, Anderson DJ, Clancy J, Crowe RR, Slymen DJ, Ghoneim MM and Hinrichs JV: Diazepam and propanolol in panic disorder and agoraphobia. *Archives of General Psychiatry* 41:287-292, 1984

Index

C

T

U

V

W

Z